# Foods That Heal
## The Natural Way to Good

*"There are illnesses that can only be treated by nutrition".*

Hippocrates

In this era of wonder drugs, hormones and synthetic compounds, it may seem an anachronism to consider therapeutics based primarily on the use of plants, vegetables, fruits and grains. But is it really so?

There are numerous disorders that can be prevented and treated by selecting natural foods rich in minerals, vitamins, trace elements, vital nutrients and other substances which have positive medicinal and curative properties.

Examples abound : The ancients knew that apple cleansed the blood, controlled high blood pressure and stimulated the flow of urine. Now, science has shown how. Apples lower sodium chloride, while increasing potassium and alkaline reserves

Recent medical research has established onion as an effective preventive food against heart attack; they correct thrombosis and reduce blood cholesterol.

Garlic juice dissolves accumulation of mucus in the sinus cavities, bronchial tubes, lungs, and reduces the severity of asthmatic attacks. Blood sugar is controlled by *amla*; it stimulates production of hormone insulin.

Scurvy resists treatment with synthetic vitamin C, yet reponds quickly to certain vegetables and fruit like cabbage, lemon and limes. The list is endless...

Lucid, easy-to-follow and devoid of medical jargon, the book is an invaluable guide for a better understanding of health, food and natural remedies. Cross indexed on foods and ailments for quick and handy reference.

*"an invaluable reference for good health".*

Dr. J.M. Jussawalla

## The Author

Mr. H.K. Bakhru enjoys a countrywide reputation as an expert on naturopathy. A prolific writer, his well-researched articles on nature cure, health and nutrition, appear regularly in various newspapers and periodicals. A diploma holder in Naturopathy, his two earlier books, Health, the Natural Way and Diet Cure for Common Ailments were highly appreciated by the public.

Mr. Bakhru, a post graduate of Lucknow University, began his career in the Indian Railways in 1949. He retired, in 1984, after 35 years of distinguished service in the Public Relations Organisation of the Indian Railways and the Railway Board, acquiring rich and varied professional experience in the field of journalism, public relations and advertising.

This book, like his earlier books, has been well-tested by his vast expertise and personal experience in the field. He has made comprehensive study of the therapeutic value of natural foods, an invaluable guide to the natural way to health, which is recorded in this book. A member of the Natural Cure Practitioners Guild in Bombay, Mr. Bakhru spends his retired life, devoting all his time to the furtherance of the cause of nature cure. His advice is always available to those who come to seek his help in the field. He may be contacted at *23, New Bombay Railwaymen's Co-op. Housing Society. Sector - 2, Vashi, New Bombay - 400 703.*

# Foods That Heal
## The Natural Way to Good Health

H.K. Bakhru

ORIENT PAPERBACKS
A Divison of Vision Books Pvt. Ltd.
New Delhi • Mumbai • Hyderabad

## Acknowledgement

"I am greatful to Dr. J.M. Jussawalla, an eminent naturopath and a member of the Governing Body of the Central Council of Research in Yoga and Naturopathy for this foreward."

ISBN 81-222-0033-8

1st Published 1990
13th Printing 1998
14th Printing 1998
15th Printing 1999

*Foods That Heal: The Natural Way to Good Health*

© H.K. Bakhru

Cover design by Vision Studio

Published by
**Orient Paperbacks**
(A division of Vision Books Pvt. Ltd.)
Madarsa Road, Kashmere Gate, Delhi-110 006

Printed in India at
Kay Kay Printers, Delhi-110 007

Cover Printed at
Ravindra Printing Press, Delhi-110 006

# Foreword

Never before has the average man and woman been better fed and so poorly nourished. The progress of civilization has led to an increasing concentration of population in cities, metropolis, and megalopolis. As a consequence man has become divorced from nature and its rich, beautiful bounty. Innumerable timeassuring, preserved, refrigerated, treated, embalmed, processed, chemicalized and pasteurized food items are being promoted with all push and vigour for merely making them commercialized. Such foods can never substitute wholesome, natural food items.

Undoubtedly, this distance from nature has denied the present generation of farm-fresh foods prepared by nature to meet man's nutritional needs. Most food, specially the increasingly popular 'convenience foods' are largely denatured, artificially flavoured, turgid and semi-synthetic; devoid of their vital food values. Whatever nutrients are left in them after long processing, storage and transportation are poor substitutes for natural "wholesomeness". Such packed and preserved foods are nothing but foodless foods.

*Foods That Heal* by H.K. Bakhru is 'Know Your Food Guide'. It will be a valuable book of reference for one and all seeking good health and prevention of ailments. This practical guide on natural foods is exhaustive study of food values, curative and natural benefits of all food items used in our day-to-day consumption.

Dr. J.M. Jussawalla
Director and President,
International Federation of the
Scientific Research Society, India;
Director, Natural Therapy Clinic, Bombay.

# Preface

"Your food shall be your medicine", said Hippocrates, father of medicine, several hundred years ago. This maxim is as relevant today. I write this from my personal experience. And this has proved to be very valid in my own case. From an early age, I was afflicted with several serious ailments. At the young age of 16, I contracted pleurisy and typhoid fever of long duration. Subsequent years saw me dogged with numerous critical ailments, including hyperacidity with severe heartburn, breathing trouble, stroke, suspected brain tumour, chronic duodenal ulcer, spondylosis, mylagia, hiatus hernia with peptic oesophageal ulcers, suspected heart disease, insomnia, backache and prostate enlargement.

The modern medical system failed to provide me any relief from these diseases and I underwent a great deal of physical suffering and mental anguish for almost 40 long years. Eventually, at the advanced age of 55, I made a determined bid to give up all drugs and take resort to the natural methods of treatment.

Diet played a decisive role in the success of this therapy. It was primarily through a selective diet of natural foods such as fresh and dried fruits, vegetables, grains, nuts, seeds and special protective foods like milk, curd and honey that I succeeded in controlling several dreaded disabilities. The experience prompted me to explore the medicinal virtues of foods in their natural form and popularise them through articles published in *The Times of India, The Economic Times* and other publications. The readers' response was overwhelming and this encouraged me to study the subject in greater depth and present it in the form of a book, which furnishes elaborate details about the use of various natural foods in the healing of specific diseases, besides other information.

H.K. Bakhru

# Contents

# Index of Diseases

## A

Acidity 46, 60, 187, 191, 210, 215

Acidosis 80, 146, 149

Acne 71

Acute digestive disorders 27

Ageing premature 50, 88, 101, 205

Alcoholism 44, 96

Allergies 33

Anaemia 19, 24, 33, 66, 81, 84, 92, 93, 111, 126, 132, 144, 146, 171, 183, 198, 201, 208

Anal itching 78, 205

Apendicitis 79, 103, 164, 176, 205

Arterisclerosis 57, 86, 93, 115, 208

Arthritis 20, 33, 64, 106, 118

Ascites 188

Asthma 33, 40, 43, 49, 71, 88, 96, 108, 115, 116, 122, 128, 147, 184, 196, 209, 213

## B

Baldness 178

Bad breath 27, 113

Beauty aids 27, 57, 62, 106, 109, 176, 192, 213

Beriberi 201

Bites, insect 62, 68, 129

Blackheads 141

Bleeding excessive 35, 89

Bleeding from nose, lung, gums etc. 89, 128, 132, 146

Blindness, night 146

Blood clotting 86

Blood circulation, poor 56, 93, 95, 165, 213

Blood disorders 65, 95

Blood pressure, high 20, 57, 117, 160

Boils 95, 119, 133, 213

Breast milk, checking secretion of 178

Breast milk deficiency 126, 147

Bright's disease 27

Bronchial congestion 108, 116, 122, 132, 140, 147, 184

Bronchitis 49, 71, 96, 108, 112, 122, 128, 132, 147, 184, 199, 201, 213

Burning of soles & heals 55, 165

Burning of rectum 205

Burns and wounds 35, 161, 165, 188, 198, 209

## C

Cancer 118, 161

Catarrah 55, 112, 174

Cholera 57, 60, 96, 106. 109. 133, 176, 187

Cholesterol, high 201

Cirrhosis of liver 74

# *Importance of Fruits in Diet*

Fruits are one of the oldest forms of food known to man. In fact, Adam, the first man ate an apple, the 'forbidden fruit' of heaven. There are many references to fruits in ancient literature. *Vedas* state that the fruits form the base of the Food of Gods. According to *Quran,* the fruits like grape, date, fig, olive and pomegranate are the gifts and heavenly fruits of God.

The people in ancient times regarded fruits to be endowed with magic,or divine properties. They gave them due reverence and dedicated them to their gods and goddesses. They also used their designs in decorating temples, vestments or ceremonial garments and sacred vessels.

Fresh and dry fruits are the natural staple food of man. They contain substantial quantities of essential nutrients in a rational proportion. They are excellent sources of minerals, vitamins and enzymes. They are easily digested and exercise a cleansing effect on the blood and the digestive tract. Persons subsisting on this natural diet will always enjoy good health. Moreover, the ailments caused by the intake of unnatural foods can be successfully treated by fruits. Fresh and dry fruits are thus not only a good food but also a good medicine.

## Natural Benefits of Fruits

Fruits have highly beneficial effect on the human system. The main physiological actions of fruits are as follows:

## Hydrating Effect

Taking of fruits or fruit juice  is the most pleasant way of hydrating the organism. The water absorbed by sick persons in this manner has an added advantage of supplying sugar and minerals at the same time.

13

## Diuretic Effect

Clinical observations have shown that potassium, magnesium and sodium contents of the fruit act as a diuretic and diuresis —frequency of urination is considerably increased when fruits and fruit juices are taken. They lower the urine density and thereby accelerate the elimination of nitrogenous waste and chlorides. As, however, fruits contain a very low level of sodium, they make a valuable contribution to a salt-free diet.

## Alkalinising Effect

The organic acids of the salts in fruits produce alkaline carbonates, when transformed within the organism, which alkalise the fluids. All fruits promote intestinal elimination. This keeps the body free from toxic wastes·which creep into the blood from an overloaded, sluggish intestinal tract. The carbohydrates of fruits are chiefly in the form of sugar, dextrin and acids which are easily digestible and are completely absorbed. Hence, they are very useful for sick and invalids for quick energy and heat.

## Mineralising Effect

Fruits furnish minerals to the body. Dried fruits such as apricots, raisins and dates are rich in calcium and iron. These minerals are essential for strong bones and good blood respectively. Some fruits, like custard apple, furnish calcium to the extent of 800 mg. per fruit, which is sufficient to meet our daily requirement of this mineral.

## Laxative Effect

The fibrous matter in fruits, cellulose, aids in the smooth passage of the food in the digestive tract and easy bowel action. The sugars and organic acids contained in fruits also increase their laxative effect. Hence, regular use of fruits prevents and cures constipation.

## Tonic Action

Fruits, as dependable sources of vitamins, exert a tonic effect in the body. Guavas, custard apples and citrus fruits, like lemons and oranges, are particularly valuable sources of vitamin C. These fruits are usually eaten fresh and raw, thus making the vitamins fully available to us. Several fruits contain good amounts of carotene which gets converted to vitamin A in the body. A medium-sized mango can provide as much as 15,000 international units of vitamin A which is sufficient for full one week and this vitamin can be stored in the body. The common papaya is an excellent source of vitamin C and carotene.

Fruits are at their best when eaten in the raw and ripe state. In cooking, they lose portions of the nutrient salts and carbohydrates. They are most beneficial when taken as a separate meal by themselves, preferably for breakfast in the morning. A combination of fruits with vegetables is not considered good. If it becomes necessary to take fruits with regular food, they should form a larger proportion of the meals. Fruits, however, make better combination with milk than with meals. It is also desirable to take one kind of fruit at a time.

In case of sickness, it will be advisable to take fruits in the form of juice. However, juice should be taken immediately after extraction as it begins to decompose quickly and loses its properties.

**Fruit Cure**

Fruits are highly beneficial in maintaining acid-alkaline balance in the body. They neutralise the toxic condition of the body resulting from excessive intake of acid-forming foods and restore its alkalinity. They help clear the system of morbid waste and cater to the body's requirement of natural sugar, vitamins and minerals.

Adolf Just, the world famous naturopath, in his book, *Return to Nature* states, "Fruits alone contain healing draughts for man; Nature offers them redymade, they taste deliciously and are sure to cure all his suffering and disease. Fruit contains nectar and ambrosia".

Fasting is considered as Nature's oldest and most effective method of treating diseases. The best and safest way of fasting is 'juice fasting'. The procedure is to take the juice of an orange or any other juicy fruits, such as grapes, grapefruit, *mosambi* and pineapple, diluted 50:50 with water, every two hours from 8 a.m. to 8 p.m. Nothing else, whatsoever, may be taken, as otherwise the value of the juice fast will be entirely lost. Canned or frozen juices should not be used. The total daily liquid intake should be about six to eight glasses.

Vitamins, minerals, enzymes and trace elements contained in fresh fruit juices are extremely beneficial in normalising all the body processes. They supply needed elements for the body's own

15

healing activity and cell regeneration and thereby speed up the recovery. Each day, while fasting it should be ensured that the bowels are cleansed of the toxic matter thrown off by the self-cleansing process set up by the body. This can be done by a warm water enema.

Next to the short juice fasting, the all-fruit diet is nature's finest eliminating medium. The value of fresh juicy fruits in overcoming of all diseased conditions, especially chronic diseases, by the cleansing of tissues, is incalculable. The all-fruit diet is highly beneficial particularly in cases of bronchitis, rheumatism, chronic catarrh and constipation as it fills the body with life-giving mineral salts.

In the case of the all-fruit diet, one should take three meals a day of fresh, ripe juicy fruits such as apples, pears, grapes, oranges, grapefruit, pineapple, peaches, melon or any other juicy fruit in season. Bananas should, however, not be taken, nor should any other foodstuff be added to the fruit diet. For drinks, plain water or unsweetened lemon water may be taken.

**Curative Properties of Fruits**

Moreover, certain fruits can combat specific ailments. It should, however, be remembered that in the therapeutic use of any fruit as a treatment for specific disease, nothing except that particular fruit or its juice should be taken in the system at the time of treatment. Thus, when utilising lemon juice as a food remedy, the juice should be taken at least half an hour before consuming any other food.

It has been found that fruit sugars, calcium, iron, vitamins A, B-complex and C control the gradation of heart energy. Hence, eating fruits like apple, lemon, orange and pomegranate can aid the proper functioning of the heart and keep it healthy even in old age. Fruits like apple, date and mango have a direct action on the central nervous system. The phosphorus, glutamic acid and vitamins A and B-complex of these fruits exert a protective and tonic effect on the nerves. Hence, regular use of these fruits in the diet will sharpen memory and prevent nervous exhaustion, mental tension, hysteria and insomnia.

All berries, being extremely rich in iron, phosphorus and sodium, are highly beneficial for blood building and nerve strengthening. The lemon can be a good food remedy in case of liver ailments, indigestion and rheumatism. Watermelons make the best kidney cleansers. The water flushes through the kidneys and the traces of various minerals contained in the water act as healing agents.

The soothing qualities of pineapple and pomegranates are helpful in catarrh, hay fever and other chronic nasal and bronchial ailments. The common cold may be treated with grapefruit juice. This juice helps rout the infection by activating the organs of elimination.

Fresh and fully ripe fruits like grapes, apples, bananas and figs are best suited for all brain deficiencies. They contain a superior quality of easily assimilable sugar which is transformed into physical energy that refreshes the brain. The kernel of walnut is a positive remedy for weakness of the brain.

A generous intake of fruits in the diet will enable a person to lead a healthy life. Fruits prevent all diseases and keep a person smart, energetic and active all through his life upto the ripe old age

# *Apple*

Botanical Name : *Malus sylvestris*
Indian Name : *Seb or Sev*

### Description

The apple is a sub-acid fruit and one of the most valuable of all the fruits It is a fleshy fruit, with tough skin, ranging in colour from greenish yellow to red. It is usually five to seven cm in diameter and has pinkish or yellowish white flesh. The apple is considered "protective" and most wholesome food. Apart from its energy value, it plays an important role in the normal development of metabolic functions—i.e. the chemical and physical changes that take place within the body and enable its continued growth and functioning

### Origin and Distribution

The apple is a native of Eastern Europe and Western Asia and has been cultivated from pre-historic times. It has mentioned in the annals of old China, Babylon and Egypt. The Bible also contains several references to this fruit. The Scandinavians called it the "Food of Gods" and believed that it possessed medicinal properties to regenerate both mind and body. In India, apples are grown in the hilly areas of Kashmir, Kulu and Kumaon. Nearly 7,500 varieties of the fruit are grown all over the world

## Food Value

The apple is a highly nutritive food. It contains minerals and vitamins in abundance. The food value of the apple is chiefly constituted by its contents of sugar which ranges from 9 to 51 per cent. Of this, fruit sugar constitutes 60 per cent and glucose 25 per cent and cane sugar only 15 per cent.

### Apple*

| Food Value | | Minerals and Vitamins | |
|---|---|---|---|
| Moisture | 84.6% | Calcium | 10 mg |
| Protein | 0.2% | Phosphorus | 14 mg |
| Fat | 0.5% | Iron | 1 mg |
| Minerals | 0.3% | Vitamin A | 40 IU** |
| Fibre | 1.0% | Small amounts of | |
| Carbohydrates | 13.4% | Vitamin E, H and | |
| | 100% | B Complex | |
| | | Calorific Value - 59 | |

*Values per 100 gms edible portion          **International Unit

Raw apples generally contain a small quantity of starch which gets wholly converted into sugar during the process of ripening. The acid content of the apple is also increased together with the sugar. This acid is constituted mostly by malic acid which is completely utilised by the body.

The skin of the apple should not be discarded when taking it in raw form as the skin and the flesh just below it contain more vitamin C than the inner flesh. The vitamin content decreases gradually towards the centre of the fruit The skin also contains five times more vitamin A than the flesh.

## Natural Benefits and Curative Properties

Apples are invaluable in the maintenance of good health and in the treatment of many ailments. It was said long ago, 'to eat an apple before going to bed will make the doctor beg his bread'. The modern version of this ancient saving, 'an apple a day keeps

18

the doctor away', sums up the healthful and nourishing qualities of apples.

The active medicinal principle of apple is pectin, natural therapeutic ingredient found in the inner portion of the rind and the pulp Pectin aids in detoxification by supplying the 'galacturonic acid' needed for the elimination of certain harmful substances It also helps to prevent decomposition of protein matter in the alimentary canal. The malic acid contained in the apple is beneficial to the bowels, liver and brain.

### Anaemia

Apples, being rich in iron, arsenic and phosphorus, are highly beneficial in the treatment of anaemia. It will be particularly useful in the form of freshly prepared apple juice. It may be taken in quantities of 1kg. daily with beneficial results. The best time to take the juice is half an hour before meals and just before retiring to bed. The cider should be drawn from selected apples which should be thoroughly washed before crushing

### Constipation and Diarrhoea

Apples are beneficial in the treatment of both constipation and diarrhoea. Raw apples are good for constipation. At least two apples should be taken daily for proper evacuation of bowels Cooked or baked apples are good for diarrhoea The cooking process softens the cellulose and provides bulk to the faeces.

### Dysentery

Apples have been found useful in acute and chronic dysentery among children. Ripe and sweet apples should be crushed into pulp and given to the child several times a day, from one to four tablespoonfuls, according to age, in this disorder The American Medical Association has also advocated the use of apples as therapeutic agent in dysentery

### Stomach Disorders

A natural 'apple medicine' for the disturbed stomach is prepared by slicing a whole apple and gently pounding it until it becomes slightly mashed. It may be sprinkled with cinnamon or honey The entire mashed apple may be eaten except for the stem and seeds It should be chewed thoroughly before swallowing This preparation should be taken several times between meals for beneficial results The all-natural medicinal substance, pectin, in the mashed apple works to create a protective coating action by virtue of its qualities as an absorbent and demulcent i.e. the soothing agent.

Shredded apple, mixed with a tablespoonful of honey and sprinkled with sesame seeds, constitute an excellent stomach tonic and an appetiser It should be taken before meals. It stimulates sluggish digestive juices and this facilitates assimilation of food for healthful results.[1]

### Headache

Apples are highly beneficial in the treatment of all types of headache. A ripe apple, after removing the upper rind and the inner hard portion should be taken with a little salt every morning on empty stomach in such cases. This should be continued for about a week. It will yield good results even in cases of disgusting chronic headache.

### Heart Disease

Apples are of special value to heart patients. They are rich in potassium and phosphorus but low in sodium. From ancient times, apple with honey is considered a very effective remedy for functional disorders of heart. Recent researches by Dr. Elizabeth Barret-Cannor of California University have revealed that people who consume plenty of potassium through food items are likely to escape heart attacks. Apples, as a good source of potassium, help in the alleviation of heart disease

### High Blood Pressure

Apples are considered invaluable in the cases of high blood pressure. The apple diet has a rapid and considerable diuretic effect causing increased secretion of urine and thus bringing down blood pressure to normal. It also relieves the kidneys by reducing the supply of sodium chloride to a minimum In addition, it lowers the sodium level in the tissues because of the high level of potassium in apples.

### Rheumatic Afflictions

Apples are regarded an excellent food medicine for gout, arthritis and rheumatism especially when these diseases are

---

1. Carlson Wade, *Health Secrets from the Orient,*pp. 62-63, Allied Publishers Pvt. Ltd., Bombay.

caused by uric acid poisoning. The malic acid contained in them is believed to neutralise the uric acid and afford relief to the sufferers. Apples, boiled to a jelly, make a very good liniment for rheumatic pains. They should be rubbed freely on the affected area

## Dry Cough

Sweet apples are valuable in dry hacking cough. Nearly 250 grams of sweet apples should be taken daily for about a week to obtain relief

## Kidney Stones

Apples are useful in kidney stones. In countries where the natural unsweetened cider is the common beverage, cases of stone or calculus are practically absent. The ripe fresh fruit will be more valuable.

## Eye Disorders

The apple peel water is an excellent medicine for the inflamed eyes both as a beverage and as an eye wash. This beverage is prepared by putting the peelings in a pan, well covered with water. The water should be brought to boiling point and allowed to simmer gently for a few minutes The water should then be strained off and some honey be added to it.[2]

The over-ripe apples are useful as a poultice for sore eyes The pulp is applied over the closed eyes and is held in position with a bandage. It is allowed to remain there for one to two hours.

## Dental Disorders

Tooth-decay can be prevented by regular consumption of apples as they possess a mouth cleansing property Dr. T.T. Hanks in his book, *Dental Survey,* says, "Apples have mouth cleansing property that no other fruit possesses, and taken after meals, they have the same effect as a tooth brush in cleansing the teeth, with the added advantage that the acid content, aside from its nutritive value, is of assistance in promoting the flow of saliva in the mouth, which is also beneficial to the teeth"[3]. The acid of the apple also exerts an antiseptic influence upon the germs

2. Eric F.W. Powell, *Health from the Kitchen,* p. 22, Health Science Press, England.

3. Dr. S.J. Singh, *Food Remedies,* p. 21, Nature Cure Council of Medical Research, Lucknow, 1982.

present in the mouth and teeth when it is thoroughly chewed. Apples are thus regarded as a natural preserver of the teeth and should be taken in all tooth troubles.

## Promotes Vigour and Vitality

The apple is the best fruit to tone up a weak and run-down condition of the human system. It removes all deficiencies of vital organs and makes the body stout and strong. It tones up the body and the brain as it contains more phosphorus and iron than any other fruit or vegetable. Its regular consumption with milk promotes health and youthfulness and helps build healthy and bright skin. It has a calming and relaxing effect and is good especially for sedentary workers.

## Uses

The apple is generally taken raw and is used as a dessert fruit. Apples can be used as a salad and taken with other fruits, or cooked or baked They can also be used in the form of dried apple, apple jelly, apple juice or cider and vinegar. Freshly prepared apple juice is one of the best fruit juices.

## Precautions

Apples should not be consumed on an empty stomach as it may lead to indigestion Apples are often sprayed with poisonous chemicals to prevent them from decay, the fruits should be thoroughly washed and cleaned in all possible ways before consumption.

# *Apricot*

Botanical Name . *Prunus armeniaca*
Indian Names : *Khubāni, Zardālu*

## Description

The apricot is one of the most important fruits. It belongs to the sub-acid class. It is somewhat acid in its raw state, but its acidity decreases and the sugar content increases in the process of ripening. The fruit is regarded as a nutritious and tonic food and enjoys world-wide popularity

The apricot is a stone fruit and has nut within it. It is round or oblong in shape, flattened to some extent. It is similar in shape as peach, but is considerably smaller. It is yellowish in colour. The fruit which ripens on the tree alone develops its true flavour which is very much like that of the peach.

**Origin and Distribution**

The apricot is believed to have originated in China, where it has been cultivated for over 4,000 years. It has also been grown in India and Tibet from time immemorial. The Hunzas, who live in the Himalayan mountains of northern Pakistan and are known for their vitality and longevity, have cultivated and valued this fruit for its health-building virtues for over 1,500 years. It was regarded as a food medicine by Greek physicians, while the Romans dedicated it to Venus, the goddess of love

It was introduced in Europe during the time of Alexander, the Great. In the Middle East, apricots were very popular for their taste as well as for their invigorating perfume.

**Food Value**

Apricots are rich in various food ingredients. The fresh fruit

### Fresh Apricot*

| Food Value | | Minerals and Vitamins | |
|---|---|---|---|
| Moisture | 85.3% | Calcium | 20 mg |
| Protein | 1.0% | Phosphorus | 25 mg |
| Fat | 0.3% | Iron | 2.2 mg |
| Minerals | 0.7% | Vitamin C | 6 mg |
| Fibre | 1.0% | Small amount of | |
| Carbohydrates | 11.6% | Vitamin B Complex | |
| | 100% | | |

**Calorific Value - 53**

### Dried Apricot*

| Food Value | | Minerals and Vitamins | |
|---|---|---|---|
| Moisture | 19.4% | Calcium | 110 mg |
| Protein | 1.6% | Phosphorus | 70 mg |
| Fat | 0.7% | Iron | 4.6 mg |
| Minerals | 2.8% | Vitamin C | 2 mg |
| Fibre | 2.1% | Small amount of | |
| Carbohydrates | 73.4% | Vitamin B Complex | |
| | 100% | | |

*Value per 100 gms edible portion    **Calorific Value - 306**

is rich in natural sugars, vitamin A and calcium. It is a good source of the Vitamins, i.e. B Complex, riboflavin and niacin as well as vitamin C. The nut of the apricot is rich in protein and fat and is considered as valuable as any other nut. It contains 40 to 45 per cent of an oil which is practically identical with almond oil in its physical as well as chemical properties

## Natural Benefits and Curative Properties

Throughout the centuries, the fruit, kernels, oil and flowers of the apricot have been used in medicine. In China, a famous medicine known as 'Apricot Gold' was made from the kernels of trees which grew in certain areas. This medicine was reputed for the powers to prolong life. The Chinese also believed that apricots reacted sympathetically to women's ailments The apricot flowers, therefore, formed a common ingredient in their cosmetics.

The kernel, which yields an oil similar to that of the almond, have been widely used for their sedative, antispasmodic that gives relief to strained muscles and demulcent or soothing properties. They are useful in the healing of wounds, in expelling worms and as a general tonic.

### Constipation

The fruit is highly valued as a gentle laxative and is beneficial in the treatment of constipation. This is due to its cellulose and pectin contents. The cellulose, which is not digested, acts as a roughage—that indigestable part of the food which helps the bowel movement and the pectin which absorbs and retains water, thereby increasing bulk to faeces and stimulating smooth bowel movement. Patients suffering from chronic constipation can greatly benefit by regular use of apricots Generally six to eight apricots used per day will produce the desired result.

### Indigestion

Apricots have an alkaline reaction in the system. They aid the digestion, if consumed before a meal. Marmalade, made from organically grown fruit, is also valuable in the treatment of nervous indigestion.

### Anaemia

The apricot is an excellent food remedy for anaemia on account of its high content of iron. The small but essential amount of copper in the fruit makes iron available to the body According to Dr. Whipple and Dr. Robschiet Robbins, the production of haemoglobin could be increased in the body by liberal use of apricots.[1]

## Fevers

Fresh juice of apricots, mixed with glucose or honey, is a very cooling drink during fevers. It quenches the thirst and eliminates the waste products from the body. It tones up the eyes, stomach, liver, heart and nerves by supplying vitamins and minerals.

## Skin Diseases

Fresh juice of apricot leaves is useful in skin diseases. It can be applied with beneficial results in scabies, eczema, sun-burn and itching of the skin due to cold exposure

## Uses

The apricot in its fresh form is used as a dessert fruit. It is, however, generally used in its dried form. The heat renders it easier to digest. It is made into excellent jam, jelly, marmalades and preserves Apricots canned in sugar are also popular The nut of the apricot is extensively used in confectionary

# *Avocado*

Botanical Name : *Persea americana*
Other English Names : *Alligator Pear, Butter Fruit*
Indian Names : *Kulu Nāspati or Mākhanphal*

## Description

The avocado is a large fleshy pear-shaped berry. It has a single large seed surrounded by buttery pulp and a hard skin. It is yellowish-green to maroon and purple in colour. The avocado tree is evergreen. It is shallow-rooted and there are no visible root hairs. It has spirally-arranged leaves, variable in shape and size and fragrant yellowish flowers.

---

1. Fairfax T. Proudfit, *Nutrition and Diet Therapy,* p. 251. Macmillan and Co., New York, 1934

## Origin and Distribution

The avocado originated in Central America. The early Spanish explorers recorded its cultivation from Mexico to Peru It was taken to southern Spain in 1601. The fruit was introduced in Mauritius in 1780 and it spread in Asia mostly in the mid-19th century. Avocados are now grown in most tropical and subtropical countries including South Africa and Australia.

## Food Value

The avocado contains more fat than any other fruit except the olive. Its fat is of the highest quality, wholly free from the unpleasant butyric acid with which many fats are contaminated. It contains a sufficient amount of vitamin A to maintain high resistance against bacterial infection, a quality possessed by few vegetable fats.

### Avocado*

| Food Value | | Minerals and Vitamins | |
|---|---|---|---|
| Moisture | 73.6% | Calcium | 10 mg |
| Protein | 1.7% | Phosphorus | 80 mg |
| Fat | 22.8% | Iron | 0.7 mg |
| Minerals | 1.1% | Vitamin A | 290 I.U |
| Carbohydrates | 0.8% | Sufficient amount of | |
| | 100% | Vitamin E and small amount of Vitamin C and Vitamin B Complex | |

*Values per 100 gms edible portion          **Calorific Value** - 215

The protein of avocado is of the finest quality and is much superior to protein of bread and other cereal foods. Its composi tion is almost identical with that of milk. In fact, the pulp of the fruit is so free from fibre that it forms, with water, a fine emul sion which closely resembles milk in consistency and appear ance. With the exception of an excess of fat and the lack of vitamin C, it may serve as a very satisfactory substitute for dairy milk. Prepared thus, the avocado may be given safely to young infants and to the feeble invalids

## Natural Benefits and Curative Properties

The avocado possesses virtues of extraordinary character. For purity, wholesomeness, ease of digestibility and adaptation to human needs, it has few rivals.

## Digestive System Disorders

The avocado is an excellent food remedy in acute digestive disorders. Its blandness is comforting to the hypersensitive surfaces of the stomach and duodenum, and its abundant vitamins reanimate the inflamed and crippled cells. The physicians in China have, for centuries, prescribed the juice of this fruit for colic and chills in the stomach. The Japanese employ the same remedy to treat ulceration of the intestines.

The avocado is an efficient aid in changing the intestinal flora to combat autointoxication, colitis, and biliousness. In cases of hyperacidity with sour stomach, avocado and well ripened papaya should be used as a staple diet. These two fruits are most appropriate foods in cases of duodenitis and duodenal ulcer, because they are bland or soothing to the sensitive membrane and pass quickly into the intestine

## Bad Breath

The avocado is far superior to any mouth lotion or remedies for bad breath. It effectively removes intestinal putrefactions or decomposition which is the real cause of a coated tongue and bad breath.

## Bright's Disease

The avocado is especially useful as a staple food in cases of Bright's disease because of its small protein content and with none of the poisonous extractives present in the flesh of this fruit.

## Psoriasis

The oil of avocado is considered beneficial in treatment of psoriasis. It should be applied gently to the affected parts. It helps in taking the scales off.

## Beauty Aid

The oil extracted from the avocado is employed in the preparation of cosmetics. A wide range of beauty aids with an avocado base are now available. These include creams, cleansers and moisturizers to prevent the ageing effect of dehydration, skin foods, bath oils, shampoos which give a rich lather and act as a scalp conditioner and revitalize dull hair

## Precaution

As avocados become sour when cooked and cannot successfully survive freezing, they should be eaten raw and as fresh as possible. If they have to be kept for a short time, they should be stored at room temperature and not in a refrigerator.

# Bael Fruit

Botanical Name : *Aegle marmelos*
Other English Names : *Stone Apple and Bengal Quince*
Indian Names : *Bel and Siriphal*

## Description

The bael occupies an important place among the indigenous fruits of India It is a woody and smooth food which is 5 to 15 cm in diameter. It has numerous seeds, which are densely covered with fibrous hairs and are embedded in a thick aromatic pulp The flesh is either eaten fresh or dried.

## Origin and Distribution

The bael tree is indigenous to India. The history of this tree has been traced to Vedic period—2000 BC - 800 BC. The mention of bael fruit has been made in *Yajur Veda*. The tree has great mythological significance, and it abounds in the vicinity of temples. It is held sacred by the Hindus and according to Hindu customs, the leaves of the tree are traditionally used as sacred offering to Lord Shiva, who is believed to live under bael tree

The bael fruit is grown throughout India as well as in Sri Lanka, Bangladesh, Pakistan, Burma, Thailand and most of the south-east Asian countries.

## Food Value

An analysis of the bael fruit shows it is rich in mineral and vitamin contents. The *sherbet* made out of this fruit has all the important nutrients and health growing ingredients. It should be thick and syrupy enough to be taken with spoon and it should be thoroughly masticated. If taken hurriedly, it may produce heaviness in the stomach. The bael fruit should also not be taken in excess at a time as excessive intake of bael may produce a sensation of heaviness in the stomach and may cause gastric discomfort.

## Bael*

| Food Value | | Minerals and Vitamins | |
|---|---|---|---|
| Moisture | 61.5% | Calcium | 85 mg |
| Protein | 1.8% | Phosphorus | 50 mg |
| Fat | 0.3% | Iron | 0.6 mg |
| Minerals | 1.7% | Vitamin C | 8 mg |
| Fibre | 2.9% | Small amount of | |
| Carbohydrates | 31.8% | Vitamin B Complex | |
| | 100% | | |

*Value per 100 gms edible portion      **Calorific Value** - 137

### Natural Benefits and Curative Properties

The bael tree is one of the most useful medicinal plants of India Its medicinal properties have been described in the ancient medical treatise in Sanskrit, *Charaka Samhita* All the parts of this tree including stem, bark, root, leaves and fruit at all stages of maturity has medicinal virtues and has been used as traditional medicine for a long time.

The fruit is of considerable medicinal value when it just begins to ripen The ripe fruit is aromatic, astringent which helps construction of skin, coolant and laxative The unripe or half-ripe fruit is astringent, digestive stomachic which improves appetite and antiscorbutic, i.e. which helps to fight scurvy caused due to vitamin C deficiency

### Constipation

Ripe bael fruit is regarded as best of all laxatives It cleans and tones up the intestines. Its regular use for two or three months helps evacuate even the old accumulated faecal matter from the bowels. For best results, it should be taken in the form of *sherbat,* which is prepared from the pulp of the ripe fruit After breaking the shell, the seeds are first removed, and contents are then taken out with a spoon and passed through a sieve Milk and little sugar may be added to make it more palatable. The pulp of the ripe fruit can also be taken from the spoon without the addition of milk or sugar About 60 gms. of the fruit will suffice for an adult

### Diarrhoea and Dysentery

The unripe or half ripe fruit is perhaps, the most effective food remedy for chronic diarrhoea and dysentery where there is no fever. Best results are obtained by the use of dried bael or its powder The bael fruit, when it is still green, is sliced and dried in the sun. The dried bael slices are reduced into powder and preserved in air-tight bottles. The unripe bael can also be baked and taken with jaggery or brown sugar

The fruit appears to have little effect in acute dysentery when there is definite sensation to defaecate but instead of significant amount of faeces, blood and mucus alone are passed The powdered drug is specially recommended in this condition. Its beneficial effect is, however, most evident when the condition has become sub-acute or chronic. After the use of the fruit in these conditions, the blood gradually disappears and the stool assume a more feculent and solid form. The mucus also disappears after continued use for some time It is also a valuable remedy for chronic dysenteric conditions characterised by alternate diarrhoea and constipation [1]

## Peptic Ulcer

An infusion of bael leaves is regarded as an effective food remedy for peptic ulcer. The leaves are soaked overnight in water This water is strained and taken as a drink in the morning The pain and discomfort are relieved when this treatment is continued for a few weeks Bael leaves are rich in tannins which reduce inflammation and help healing of ulcers. The bael fruit taken in the form of beverage has also great healing properties on account of its mucliage, i e sticky or viscous content This substance forms a coating on the stomach mucosa and thus helps in the healing of ulcers.

## Respiratory Affections

A medicated oil prepared from bael leaves gives relief from recurrent colds and respiratory affections. The juice extracted from bael leaves is mixed with equal quantity of sesame oil and heated thoroughly A few seeds of black pepper and half a teaspoonful of black cumin are added to the hot oil It is then removed from the fire and stored for use when necessary A teaspoonful of this oil should be massaged into the scalp before a head bath Its regular use builds up resistance against colds and coughs

A common practice in south India is to give the juice of bael

1. Col. Chopra, *Indigenous Drugs of India*, p. 269, Academic Publishers, Calcutta, 1982.

leaves to bring relief from wheezing and respiratory spasm. The leaf juice, mixed in warm water with a little pepper, is given as a drink.

# Banana

Botanical Name : *Musa paradisiaca*
Indian Name : *Kelā*

## Description

The banana is one of the oldest and best known fruits of the world. It is delicious and seedless and is available in all seasons at a price which is within everybody's reach. It is a very hygienic fruit as it comes in a germ-proof package. Its thick covering provides an excellent protection against bacteria and contamination. The mature fruits vary in sizes and may be greenish, yellow or reddish in colour.

## Origin and Distribution

Original home of banana is believed to be India and Malaya. The fruit as well as its plant is considered to be a very auspicious in all the religious and social ceremonies in India. In the mythological ages in Europe it was called the 'apple of paradise'. The Greek and Arabian writers referred to it as a wonderful fruit of India. The Malayan soldiers probably took them to Madagascar about the fifth century AD and from there it spread to east coast and mainland of Africa. Later, it was introduced in Western countries and other parts of the world. In India, there are three important banana-producing areas South India, Western India and Eastern India from Bihar to Assam.

## Food Value

The banana is of great nutritional value. It has a rare combination of energy value, tissue-building elements, protein, vitamins and minerals. It is a good source of calories being richer in solids and lower in water content than any other fresh fruit. A large banana supplies more than 100 calories. It contains a large amount of easily assimilable sugar, making it a good source of

31

quick energy and an excellent means of recovery from fatigue.

### Banana*

| Food Value | | Minerals and Vitamins | |
|---|---|---|---|
| Moisture | 70.1% | Calcium | 17 mg |
| Protein | 1.2% | Phosphorus | 36 mg |
| Fat | 0.3% | Iron | 0.9 mg |
| Minerals | 0.8% | Vitamin C | 7 mg |
| Fibre | 0.4% | Small amount of | |
| Carbohydrates | 27.2% | Vitamin B Complex | |
| | 100% | | |

*Value per 100 gms edible portion          **Calorific Value** - 116

The banana constitutes almost a complete balanced diet in combination with milk. It contains a high grade protein, which includes three of the essential amino acids. Banana and milk supplement each other in an ideal manner and provide all the needed nutrients to the body

## Natural Benefits and Curative Properties

In the traditional medicine of India and the ancient Persia this golden fruit is regarded as nature's secret of perpetual youth. To this day, banana is known for promoting healthy digestion and creating a feeling of youthfulness. They help promote the retention of calcium, phosphorus and nitrogen—all of which then work to build sound and regenerated tissues  Banana also contains invert sugar, which is an aid to youthful growth and metabolism

### Intestinal Disorder

The banana is used as a dietary food against intestinal disorders because of its soft texture and blandness. It is said to contain an unidentified compound called, perhaps jokingly, 'vitamin U' (against ulcer). It is the only raw fruit which can be eaten without distress in chronic ulcer cases  It neutralises the over-acidity of the gastric juices and reduces the irritation of the ulcer by coating the lining of the stomach

Ripe bananas are highly beneficial in the treatment of ulcerative colitis, being bland, smooth, easily-digestible and slightly laxative  They relieve acute symptoms and promote the healing process

## Constipation and Diarrhoea

Bananas are of great value both in constipation and diarrhoea as they normalise colonic functions in the large intestine to absorb large amounts of water for proper bowel moments. Their usefulness in constipation is due to their richness in pectin, which is water-absorbent and this gives them a bulk-producing ability. They also possess the ability to change the bacteria in the intestines—from the harmful type of bacilli to the beneficial acidophyllus bacilli.

## Dysentery

Mashed banana together with little salt is a very valuable remedy for dysentery. According to Dr. Kirticar, a combination of ripe plantain, tamarind and common salt is most effective in this disease. He claims to have cured several cases of both acute and chronic dysentery by this treatment.[1] Ripe bananas are also very useful in dysentery of children, but they should be thoroughly mashed and beaten to cream before use in these cases

## Arthritis and Gout

Bananas are useful in the treatment of arthritis and gout. A diet of bananas only for three or four days is advised in these conditions. The patient can be given to eat eight or nine bananas daily during this period and nothing else.

## Anaemia

Being high in iron content, bananas are beneficial in the treatment of anaemia. They stimulate the production of haemoglobin in the blood

## Allergies

The fruit is very useful for those who are allergic to certain foods and who suffer in consequence from skin rashes or digestive disorders or asthma. Unlike other protein foods, many of which contain an amino-acid which these persons cannot tolerate and which causes allergy. Bananas contain only benign amino-acids which in most cases are not allergic. The fruit, however, does cause allergic reactions in certain sensitive persons and they should avoid it.

## Kidney Disorders

Bananas are valuable in kidney disorder because of their low

---

1. Lt. Col. Kirticar and Major R.D. Basu, *Indian Medical Plants* p. 1268, Allahabad, 1918.

protein and salt content and high carbohydrate content. They are useful in uraemia, a toxic condition of the blood due to kidney congestion and dysfunction. In such cases, a diet of bananas should only be taken for three to four days, consuming eight to nine bananas a day. This diet is suitable for all kidney troubles, including nephritis.

**Tuberculosis**

Bananas are considered useful in the treatment of tuberculosis. According to Dr. J. Montelvz of Brazil, South America, the juice of the plantain or the ordinary cooked bananas works miracles in the cure of tuberculosis. He claims to have cured patients with advanced stage of tuberculosis with frequent cough, abundant expectoration or phlegm and high fever in two months by this treatment.[2]

**Urinary Disorders**

Juice from Banana stem is a well-known remedy for urinary disorders. It improves the functional efficiency of kidney and liver thereby alleviating the discomforts and diseased condition in them. It clears the excretionory organs in the abdominal region of toxins and helps to eliminate them in the form of urine. It has been found to be of great help in the treatment for the removal of stones in the kidney, gall bladder, and prostate. It is advisable to mix this juice whenever possible with the juice of ash pumpkin.

**Over-weight**

A diet consisting of bananas and skimmed milk is considered an effective remedy for weight reduction. In prescribed course of diet treatment, the daily diet is restricted to six bananas and four glasses of skimmed milk or buttermilk made from skimmed milk for a period of 10 to 15 days. Thereafter green vegetables may be introduced gradually, reducing the intake of bananas from six to four. This regimen or prescribed course of diet treatment can be continued till the desired results are achieved. Bananas are suitable for overweight people as they contain practically no sodium.

**Menstrual Disorders**

Cooked banana flower eaten with curd is considered an

2. Dr. S.J. Singh, *Food Remedies* p. 42, Nature Cure Council of Medical Research, Lucknow, 1982.

effective medicine for menstural disorders like painful menstruation and excessive bleeding. Banana flower helps increase progestrone hormone which reduces the bleeding [3]

## Burns and Wounds

A plaster is prepared by beating a ripe banana into a fine paste. It can be spread over burns and wounds and supported by a cloth bandage. It gives immediate relief. The young tender leaves of banana tree form a cool dressing for inflammations and blisters.

## Uses

Ripe bananas are chiefly eaten raw as a dessert or a breakfast fruit. It is also used in salad together with other fruits and vegetables Unripe fruits are cooked. Banana chips are made from fully mature unripe fruits. The flour prepared from the dried unripe bananas is three times richer in minerals than the wheat flour. It is also more digestible than cereal starches and is an ideal food for infants and invalids.

## Precautions

Banana, taken as a table fruit, must be thoroughly ripe as otherwise it may be difficult to digest The raw bananas contain 20 to 25 per cent starch. But during the process of ripening, this starch is almost wholly converted with assimilable sugar

Bananas should never be kept in a refrigerator as low temperature prevents their ripening. The fruit should not be taken by those who are suffering from kidney failure because of its high potassium content.

# *Date*

Botanical Name : *Phoenix dactylifera*
Indian Name : *Khajur*

## Description

The date is one of the most nourishing fruits. It is a food of

---

3. Dr. Aman, *Medical Secrets of Your Foods*, p. 190, Indo-American Hospital, Mysore, 1985

great importance and is called the bread of the Sahara. But its use is now universal. It is included in the categories of both dry and fresh fruit The date is a cylindrical fruit of yellow to reddish brown colour. It has fleshy pericarp surrounding a single seed containing 60 to 70 per cent sugar. The tree-ripe fresh date is delicious fruit. It, however, undergoes fermentation very rapidly. It is, therefore, dried in the sun. The fruit looses about 35 per cent of its weight in the process of drying.

## Origin and Distribution

The date is held in high esteem from ancient times and is one of the earliest fruits cultivated by man. In Mesopotamia, more than 5,000 years old bricks have been found to contain instructions for growing date palms. The ancient monuments of Egypt have been found to contain carved figures of date palms There are numerous references to the palm and its fruit in the Bible, testifying to its manifold virtues Prophet Mohammed believed that the first date palm was made from the tempered dust which remained after the formation of Adam.

The original home of date is believed to be in the Persian Gulf area or in Mesopotamia. It is now classed as one of the standard crops of world agriculture and is widely grown in Saudi Arabia, Egypt, Iran, Iraq, Spain, Italy, China and U.S.A.

## Food Value

The date is a food of high nutritional value. It provides natural sugar in the form of glucose and fructose. This sugar is ready for immediate absorption and is, therefore, infinitely superior to cane-sugar. It is usually taken raw or with milk, which makes it highly nutritious in most respects. Taking it with curdled milk is also common. In Sahara, rich people take it

### Date*

| Food Value | | Minerals and Vitamins | |
|---|---|---|---|
| Moisture | 15.3% | Calcium | 120 mg |
| Protein | 2.5% | Phosphorus | 50 mg |
| Fat | 0.4% | Iron | 7.3 mg |
| Minerals | 2.1% | Vitamin C | 3 mg |
| Fibre | 3.9% | Little amount of | |
| Carbohydrates | 75.8% | Vitamin B complex | |
| | 100% | | |

*Value per 100 gms edible portion      **Calorific Value** - 317

with butter by removing the seed and filling the cavity with butter. It is a scientific way of taking fat. It is also taken in several cooked forms. The seeds of the fruit, roasted and ground into powder makes a beverage like coffee, called 'date coffee'. The date palm yields a sweet juice of high food value. It can be taken fresh with great advantage or make into a tasty country sugar The juice can also be allowed to ferment and made into alcohol

## Natural Benefits and Curative Properties

Dates are valuable as medicine for their tonic effect. Being easily digested, they are very useful for supplying energy and repairing waste. Milk in which clean and fresh dates have been boiled is a very nourishing and restorative drink to children and adults alike, especially during convalescence.

### Intestinal Disturbances

The nicotinic content in dates is an excellent remedy for intestinal disturbances. According to Metchnikoff, the great Russian scientist, liberal use of dates keeps in check the growth of pathological oragnisms and helps to establish a colony of friendly bacteria in the intestines.[1]

### Constipation

The date is a laxative food. It is highly beneficial in the treatment of constipation as the roughage provided by it stimulates sluggish bowels. They should be immersed in water at night and taken after making them into a fine syrup the next morning to secure laxative effect.

### Intoxication

Dates are an excellent remedy for alcoholic intoxication. In such cases, drinking water in which fresh dates have been rubbed or soaked will bring quick relief.

### Weak Heart

Dates are an effective remedy for weak heart. Dates soaked overnight in water and crushed in the same water in the morning after removing the seeds should be taken at least twice a week in this condition. It will strengthen the heart.

### Sexual Debility

Dates are highly beneficial in the treatment of sexual

1. K.R. Mukherjee, *Protective Foods in Health and Disease* p.53, Prakritik Chikitsalaya, Culcatta, 4th edition, 1983

weakress. A handful of dates soaked in fresh goat's milk overnight should be ground in the same milk in the morning. A pinch of cardamom powder and honey should be mixed in this preparation. This becomes a very useful tonic for improving sex stamina and sterility due to functional disorders.[2]

### Children's Diseases

According to Dr. Aman, a date tied to the wrist of the baby and allowed to be sucked by him during teething time hardens the gums and prevents other complaints like fretfulness and diarrhoea A teaspoonful of paste of the date prepared with honey is an effective medicine for diarrhoea and dysentery during teething. It should be given three times a day [3]

### Precautions

The dates require great care for selection. The sticky surface of the date attracts dust and impurities of the air to settle there. It is, therefore, advisable to purchase the best varieties in good packing condition and to wash them thoroughly before use.

# *Fig*

Botanical Name : *Ficus carica*
Indian Name : *Anjeer*

### Description

The fig occupies a high position among fruits. Soft, sweet and puply, this delicious fruit promotes health. It is a pear-shaped hollow fruit, with sugary pulp and a large number of small seeds of golden colour sticking to the wall of the cavity. It is variable in size and colour. The ripe fresh fruit is juicy, wholesome and delicious. However, being highly perishable, it is sold in the world markets in its dry form.

### Origin and Distribution

The fig is a native of Asia Minor and spread early to the Mediterranean region. It is a plant of extremely ancient

2. Dr. Aman, *Medicinal Secrets of Your Food*, p. 201, Indo American Hospital, Mysore, 1985
3. Ibid., p. 202.

cultivation and was grown in Egypt a[...]
used as a principal food in the Med[...]
thousands of years. The main areas of fig cu[...]
Pune in Maharashtra, Srirangapatnam in Kar[...]
in Uttar Pradesh and parts of Gujarat.

**Food Value**

An analysis of the fresh fig shows it consists good amo[...]
moisture and little protein, fat and carbohydrate. The dry fig [...]
a high nutritive value. Its most important food element is sugar[...]
which forms 51 to 74 per cent of the whole fruit. It can be taken in
various ways, either by itself or in combination with other
foodstuffs enrich their food value. When taken with white flour,
it removes much of its constipating effect. It combines very well
with milk. Figs are often used for preparing cakes and jams.
They are also made into pudding

## Fig* (Fresh)

| Food Value | | Minerals and Vitamins | |
|---|---|---|---|
| Moisture | 88.1% | Calcium | 35 mg |
| Protein | 1.3% | Phosphorus | 22 mg |
| Fat | 0.2% | Iron | 0.6 mg |
| Carbohydrates | 7.6% | Vitamin A | 80 IU |
| Fibre | 2.2% | Vitamin C | 2 mg |
| Minerals | 0.6% | Small amount of | |
| | 100% | Vitamin B Complex | |
| | | **Calorific Value - 80** | |

## Fig* (Dry)

| Food Value | | Minerals and Vitamins | |
|---|---|---|---|
| Moisture | 23.0% | Calcium | 126 mg |
| Protein | 4.3% | Phosphorus | 77 mg |
| Fat | 1.3% | Iron | 3 mg |
| Carbohydrates | 63.4% | Vitamin A | 80 IU |
| Fibre | 5.6% | Small amount of | |
| Minerals | 2.4% | Vitamin B Complex | |
| | 100% | | |

*Value per 100 gms edible portion          **Calorific Value - 274**

## Natural Benefits and Curative Properties

Many medicinal virtues have been ascribed to the fig. It is
considered a restorative food which helps in quick recovery after

cal and mental exertion and
gour and strength. It is an
le who suffer cracks in lips,

d, the fig is regarded as a
of its large cellulose content and
the fruit possess the property of
like movements of intestines
tion of faeces and keeps the

erty, the fig is an excellent remedy
for piles. Figs should be soaked in cold water
in a glass of enamelware in the night after cleaning them
thoroughly with hot water. They should be taken next morning.
Figs should be taken similarly in the evening. This will remove
straining at stools and thus prevent the protrusion of the anus.
The piles will be cured with regular use of figs in this manner for
three or four weeks.

### Asthma

Figs are considered beneficial in the treatment of asthma.
Phlegmatic cases of cough and asthma are treated with success
by their use. It gives comfort to the patient by draining of the
phelgm.

### Sexual Weakness

Figs can be beneficially used in the treatment of sexual
debility. They can be supplemented by other dry fruits like
almonds and dry dates along with butter. Their use has proved
effective in such cases

### Corns

For corns of long duration, the milky juice of green figs helps
to soften them. The milk has a mild necrotic action

### Precautions

Figs should be washed thoroughly before use. The skin of the
dry fruit being tough, the soaked fig is easy to digest. It is,
however, essential to take the water along with the fruit as much
of the nutrients come out into the water.

# *Grapes*

Botanical Name : *Vitis vinifera*
Indian Name : *Angoor*

## Description

Grapes are one of the most valuable fruits, They are delicious, highly nutritious and most easily digestible. They are one of Nature's precious gifts for the revitalization of the human system.

Spherical or ovoid in shape, the grape is a form of berry. They are of innumerable varieties differing in size, shape, colour, aroma and taste. The sizes vary from as big as plums to as small as peas. They are found in various colours such as green, black, red and blue.

## Origin and Distribution

Grapes have been cultivated from time immemorial and they are one of the earliest fruit vines cultivated by man. The 8000 year old monuments of Egypt contain carvings of grapes in stone. The grape is believed to be indigenous to Caucasia and its surrounding areas. From here it gradually spread to Western Asia, Southern Europe, Algeria and Morocco. It came to India at a very early time. The main centres of grape cultivation in India are in Tamil Nadu, Nasik, Pune and Aurangabad in Maharashtra, Hyderabad in Andhra Pradesh and Punjab and Haryana. The plant grows all through the year in Hyderabad and South India.

## Food Value

The grape is a highly valued fruit mainly for its rich content

### Grapes*

| Food Value | | Minerals and Vitamins | |
|---|---|---|---|
| Moisture | 92.0% | Calcium | 20 mg |
| Protein | 0.7% | Phosphorus | 20 mg |
| Fat | 0.1% | Iron | 0.2 mg |
| Minerals | 0.2% | Vitamin C | 31 mg |
| Carbohydrates | 7.0% | Small amount of | |
| | 100% | Vitamin B Complex, | |
| | | Vitamin A and P | |

*Value per 100 gms edible portion          **Calorific Value** - 32

of sugar which is formed almost entirely by glucose. The quantity of glucose in grapes varies from 15 to 25 per cent in different varieties. The glucose is a predigested food and is absorbed in the body soon after its consumption. It supplies heat and energy to the body within a short time.

## Natural Benefits and Curative Properties

The therapeutic value of grapes is closely linked with its richness in pure glucose. Studies have indicated that the production of energy essential for the proper functioning of the heart and organs of high physiological importance depends on the metabolism of glucose. Grapes, therefore, have a restorative effect by virtue of their easy assimilation. They are thus highly valuable in case of weak digestion, general debility and fever.

The 'grape cure' is perhaps the best of the various fruit cures proposed from time to time. It consists of eating an exclusive diet of grapes daily It is an old established mode of treatment. As far back as 1556, books on this wonderful method of natural treatment had been published in the various languages of Europe. They deal with the grape cure as a remedy for various diseases. Over a hundred years ago, Dr. Lambe, a pioneer reformer and dietitian, treated cancer in England with grapes Germany seems to be the centre of this natural healing cult.

The grape diet is recommended by Dr. Herman Rieder, a university Professor, and Dr. Martin Zeller, both of Munchen, Germany For a complete cure these doctors prescribe the juice extracted from fresh grapes to be taken in five meals daily. The treatment lasts from four to six weeks and the best time for this is during September and October. In some cases large quantities of juice are administered—from 1 to 6.5 Kg. of pressed grapes being used daily [1]

## Constipation

The combination of the properties of the cellulose, sugar and organic acid in the grape makes it a laxative food. It is highly valuable in relieving constipation. Its field of action is not limited in clearing the bowels only. It tones up the stomach and intestines and relieves the most chronic cases of constipation One should take atleast 350 grams of grapes daily to achieve the

---

1. Johanna Brandt, *The Grape Cure*,pp. 147-148, Ehret Literature Publishing Co., California.

desired results. When fresh grapes are not available, raisins soaked in water can be used.

## Dyspepsia

Grapes are valuable in dyspepsia. They constitute a light food which removes indigestion and irritation of the stomach in a short time and relieves heat.

## Asthma

Grapes are considered useful in asthma. According to Dr. Oldfield, grapes and their juices are beneficial in the treatment of asthma. He thinks that the patient can recover early if he is kept in a garden of grapes.[2]

## Heart Disease

Grapes are highly beneficial in the treatment of heart disease. They tone up the heart and are effective in cardiac pain and palpitation of the heart. The diseases can be rapidly controlled if the patient adopts an exclusive grape diet for few days. Grape juice will be valuable when one is actually suffering from a heart attack. This will avert serious consequences by reducing the pain and palpitation.

## Migraine

The juice of ripe grapes is a very effective home remedy for migraine. It is said that King Jamshed, who was very fond of grapes, once stored the juice of grapes well packed in bottles and made it public that the bottles contained strong poison so as to prevent others from taking it. It so happened that the wife of the king was struck with migraine and having obtained no relief from any treatment, decided to end her life by taking this so called 'poison' She took it several times in small doses and contrary to her expectations, it gave her great relief instead of killing her.[3]

## Kidney Troubles

The grape has an exceptional diuretic value on account of its high contents of water and potassium salt. Its value in kidney troubles is enhanced by its low albumin and sodium chloride content. It is an excellent food remedy in acute and chronic nepthritis and in kidney and bladder stones.

2. Kvj. Ganpati Singh Verma, *Miracles of Fruits*, p. 23, The Rasayan Pharmacy, New Delhi, 9th Edition 1978.

3. Ibid p. 5

## Liver Disorders

Grapes activate the liver or hepatic functions to stimulate glycogenic functions and bile secretion They are thus highly beneficial in the treatment of all liver disorders.

## Children's Diseases

Grape juice is excellent blood-builder. It is an effective household remedy and can be preserved in bottles. It is valuable to children in the treatment of constipation and also in the prevention of convulsions due to constipation. The juice is an effective food remedy for infants during teething trouble.

## External Sores

Grape poultices have been found effective in case of external growths, where there is an open sore. The poultice is prepared by crushing grapes and spreading them between layers of cheese cloth or muslin It should be placed over the affected parts and covered with a dry cloth The poultice should be renewed frequently as it absorbs much of the toxins.[4]

## Pyorrhoea

The organic acids of the grapes are strongly antiseptic and their effect on the gums is very effective According to Johánna Brandt, "Every tooth may be loose in its socket and pus may be pouring from the gums, but after a few weeks on the exclusive grape diet it will in time be found that the teeth are firmly set in the jaws and that every trace of pyorrhoea poisoning has disappeared"

## Alcoholism

Grapes are highly beneficial in the treatment of alcoholism. It is a very effective remedy for those craving for alcoholic drinks as it supplies the purest form of the alcohol. Grapes should form an exclusive diet in treating the alcoholics

## Precautions

Grapes have a poor keeping quality They undergo quick putrefaction. They should, therefore, be used soon after purchase or else be preserved in cold storage. While purchasing grapes, care should be taken to ensure that they are fully ripe.

---

4. Johanna Brandt, *The Grape Cure*, p.89, Ehret Literature Publishing Co., California.

# Grapefruit

Botanical Name : *Citrus paradisi*
Indian Name : *Chakotrā*

## Description

The grapefruit occupies a high place among the citrus fruits because of its flavour, its appetising properties and its refreshing qualities. The fruit is often very large—larger than the human head It varies in colour and may have a pale yellow or pinkish flesh. The rind is usually quarter to half an inch thick

## Origin and Distribution

The grapefruit is indigenous to Indo-China, Thailand and Malaya It has spread to other hot countries from these lands. It is now extensively grown in West Indies, Israel, Brazil, South Africa, Australia, Newzealand, U.S.A. and India.

## Food Value

The fruit is nutritive and refrigerant and possesses very much the same properties as the orange, lemon and lime. The seedless variety is the best as it often contains greater amount of sugar, calcium and phosphorus. The grapefruit is often used as table salad and is taken together with other fruit and vegetables. It is sometimes cut into half, and the seeds and the hard pith removed from the centre. The cavity is then filled with sugar which is also sprinkled over the cut surface. It is left for one hour in a covered plate and then taken

### Grapefruit*

| Food Value | | Minerals and Vitamins | |
|---|---|---|---|
| Moisture | 92.0% | Calcium | 20 mg |
| Protein | 0.7% | Phosphorus. | 20 mg |
| Fat | 0.1% | Iron | 0.2 mg |
| Minerals | 0.2% | Vitamin C | 31 mg |
| Carbohydrates | 7.0% | Small amount of | |
| | | Vitamins B Complex, | |
| | 100% | A and P | |
| *Value per 100 gms edible portion | | **Calorific Value** - 32 | |

## Natural Benefits and Curative Properties

The grapefruit is an excellent appetiser. It promotes salivary and gastric digestion. It is an important health-builder and a tonic.

## Acidity

Inspite of its often sharp, sub-acid taste, the fresh grapefruit has an alkaline reaction after digestion. The citric acid of the fruit is oxidized in the human system and hence the effect is to increase the alkalinity of the fluids of the body. Its juice is beneficial in the prevention and treatment of acidity and many diseases caused by too much acid in the system.

## Digestive Disorders

The fruit is valuable in relieving constipation. The pulp, when wholly taken, supplies healthy bulk to aid bowel action. It is beneficial in maintaining the health of intestines and is regarded as a preventive food item against dysentery, diarrhoea, enteritis, typhus and other infective diseases of the digestive tract.

## Diabetes

According to Dr. Joe Shelby Riley, a well-known expert in nutrition, "Grapefruit is a splendid thing in the food of diabetic patient. If grapefruits were eaten more liberally, there would be much less diabetes. If you have sugar, use three grapefruits three times a day. If you do not have sugar, but a tendency towards it and want to prevent it, use three a day Decrease starches, sweets and fats Eat mostly fruits and vegetables and juices. In two weeks this will eliminate sugar when not taking insulin. When taking insulin, it takes longer."[1]

## Influenza

The juice of grapefruit is an excellent remedy for influenza as it helps to reduce acidity in the system and its bitter properties arising from a substance called 'maringin, tones up the system and the digestive tract

## Fever

The juice of grapefruit is also an excellent diet in all fevers. It quenches thirst and removes the burning sensation produced by the fever. It should be taken mixed with water.

## Malaria

The grapefruit contains a natural 'quinine' and hence is

---

1 Dr. S.J. Singh, *Food Remedies,*p 103, Nature Cure Council of Medical Research, Lucknow, 1982.

valuable in the treatment of malaria. This 'quinine' is also beneficial in feverish colds. It can be extracted from the fruits by boiling a quarter of a grapefruit and straining the pulp.[2]

### Fatigue

The grapefruit is beneficial in the treatment of fatigue. Taking a glass of grapefruit and lemon juice in equal parts is an excellent way of dispelling fatigue and general tiredness after a day's work.

### Scanty Urination

The juice of grapefruit is extremely rich in vitamin C and potassium. It can, therefore, be beneficially used as a medicine in scanty urination caused by liver, kidney and heart disorders

# Indian Gooseberry

Botanical Name : *Emblica officinalis*
Other English Names: *Emblica myrobalan*
Indian Name : *Amlā*

### Description

Indian gooseberry is a wonderful fruit and one of the precious gifts of nature to man. It is probably the richest known natural source of vitamin C which is readily assimilated by the human system. It contributes greatly towards health and longevity

Indian gooseberry is globular small, round, six-lobed fruit, thick and hard in consistency. It is light yellow in colour and is about 1.25 cm. to 2.5 cm. in diameter.

### Origin Distribution

The Indian gooseberry is indigenous to India. It has been used as a valuable ingredient of various medicines in India and the Middle East from time immemorial. Shusrut, the great Ayurvedic authority, considers it as the best of all acid fruit and most useful in health and disease. Like Ayurvedic physicians,

---

2. Helen Jeans, *About Tropical Fruits*, p.32, Thorsons Publishers Limited, London 1972.

Hakims of Unani medicine also use it very commonly and regard it as a good medicine for heart and bodily defects. They also use it in external applications due to its cool and astringent properties.

The Indian gooseberry is grown as a commercial crop primarily in Uttar Pradesh. It also grows wild at the foot of the Himalayas and at elevation upto 1,500 metres in South India. The tree flowers in the spring and fruit ripens in the winter.

**Food Value**

Indian gooseberry is valued chiefly for its high vitamin C content. The vitamin C Value of *amla* increases further when the juice is extracted from the fruit. The dehydrated berry provides 2428 to 3470 mg. of vitamin C per 100 grams. Even when it is dried in the shade and then turned into powder, it retains as much as 1780 to 2660 mgs. of Vitamin C.

**Indian Gooseberry\***

| Food Value | | Minerals and Vitamins | |
|---|---|---|---|
| Moisture | 81.8% | Calcium | 50 mg |
| Protein | 0.5% | Phosphorus | 20 mg |
| Fat | 0.1% | Iron | 1.2 mg |
| Minerals | 0.5% | Vitamin C | 600 mg |
| Fibre | 3.4% | Small amounts of | |
| Carbohydrates | 13.7% | Vitamin B Complex | |
| | 100% | | |
| *Value per 100 gms edible portion | | **Calorific Value -48** | |

The best way to take it, with the least loss of vitamin C is to eat it raw with a little salt. The berry may also be used as a vegetable. It is often used in the form of pickles and marmalade. It can be preserved for a long period when it is dried and turned into powder

## Natural Benefits and Curative Properties

Many medicinal virtues have been attributed to Indian gooseberry. The fresh fruit is light, laxative and diuretic. A tablespoonful each of fresh gooseberry juice and honey mixed together forms a very valuable medicine for the treatment of several ailments. It should be taken every morning. Its regular use will promote vigour in the body within a few days. When fresh fruit is not available, dry powder can be mixed with honey

**Respiratory Disorders**

This medicinal tonic is highly beneficial in the treatment of respiratory disorders. It is especially valuable in tuberculosis of the lungs, asthma and bronchitis.

**Diabetes**

Indian gooseberry, with its high vitamin C content, is considered valuable in diabetes. A tablespoonful of its juice, mixed with a cup of fresh bitter gourd juice, taken daily for two months will stimulate the islets of Lengerhans i.e.—the isolated group of cells that the secrete hormone insulin. It thus reduces the blood sugar in diabetes. Diet restrictions should be strictly observed while taking this medicine. It will also prevent eye complications in diabetes.[1]

Equal quantity of *amla* powder, *jamun* powder and bitter-gourd powder also make a very useful food remedy for diabetics. A teaspoonful of this mixture once or twice a day would be effective in checking the progress of the disease.

**Heart Disease**

Indian gooseberry is considered an effective remedy for heart disease. It tones up the functions of all the organs of the body and builds up health by destroying the heterogenous elements and renewing the body energy.

**Eye Disorders**

The juice of Indian gooseberry, mixed with honey, is useful in preserving eye sight. It will also be beneficial in the treatment of conjunctivitis and glucoma. It reduces intraocular tension in a remarkable maner. A cupful of this juice should be taken mixed with honey twice daily in such cases.

**Rheumatism**

The Indian gooseberry is useful in the treatment of rheumatism. One teaspoonful of powder of the dry fruit mixed with two teaspoonfuls of jaggery should be taken twice daily for a month in this disease.[2]

**Scurvy**

As an extremely rich source of vitamin C. Indian gooseberry

1. Dr. Aman, *Medical Secrets of Your Food,* p. 399, Indo American Hospital, Mysore, 1985.
2. Ibid.,p. 400.

is one of the best remedies for scurvy. Powder of dry gooseberry mixed with equal quantity of sugar should be taken in doses of one teaspoonful three times daily with milk.

### Diarrhoea and Dysentery

The dried fruit is valuable in diarrhoea and dysentery. A drink made from *amla* mixed with lemon juice and *misri* is considered highly beneficial in controlling acute bacillary dysentery. One tablespoonful of the paste of leaves mixed with honey or butter-milk also makes an effective medicine in the treatment of diarrhoea and dysentery.

### Prevents Ageing

Indian gooseberry has revitalising effects. It contains an element which is very valuable in preventing ageing and in maintaining strength in old age. It improves body resistance and protects against infection. It strengthens the heart, hair and different glands in the body. It is said that the great ancient sage Muni Chyawan rejuvenated himself in his late 70s and regained his virility by the use of *amla*.

### Hair Tonic

Indian gooseberry is an accepted hair tonic in traditional recipes for enriching hair growth and hair pigmentation. The fruit, cut into pieces, is dried preferably in shade. These pieces are boiled in coconut oil till the solid matter becomes like charred dust. This darkish oil is an excellent oil to prevent greying. The water in which dired amla pieces are soaked overnight is also nourishing to hair. This water should be used for the last rinse while washing the hair.[3]

# *Jambul Fruit*

Botanical Name : *Syzygium cumini or Eugenia jambolana*
Other English Names : *Rose apple, Java plum*
Indian Name : *Jāmun*

### Description

The jambul fruit is a well-known common fruit. It has two

3. Dr. Girija Khanna, *Herbal Remedies*, p. 127, Tarang Paperbacks, New Delhi, 1982.

varieties. The big one is oval in shape and is commonly called as *Suva-jamun*. The small one is round in shape and is commonly called as *Kutta-jamun*. The bigger variety is sweeter than the smaller one.

The fruit is a juicy berry with a single stone. It is black outside and violet inside; has a sourish-sweet pulp and greenish yellow seed.

**Origin and Distribution**

The jambul fruit has been cultivated in the Indo-Malaysian region for a long time. It is considered to be native of India or further east, but is now found in all tropical regions and grows abundantly during the rainy season. It is a common tree, found wild or cultivated in most parts of India.

## Jambul Fruit*

| Food Value | | Minerals and Vitamins | |
|---|---|---|---|
| Moisture | 83.7% | Calcium | 15 mg |
| Protein | 0.7% | Phosphorus | 15 mg |
| Fat | 0.3% | Iron | 1.2 mg |
| Minerals | 0.4% | Vitamin C | 18 mg |
| Fibre | 0.9% | Small amount of | |
| Carbohydrates | 14.0% | Vitamin B Complex | |
| | 100% | | |

*Value per 100 gms edible portion          **Calorific Value - 62**

# Natural Benefits and Curative Properties

### Diabetes

The jambul fruit is regarded in traditional medicine as a specific against diabetes because of its effect on the pancreas. The fruit as such, the seeds and fruit juice are all useful in the treatment of this disease. The seeds contain a glucose 'Jamboline' which is believed to have the power to check the pathological conversion of starch into sugar in cases of increased production of glucose. They are dried and powdered. This powder in doses of three grams should be given three or four times a day mixed in water. It reduces the quantity of sugar in urine and allays the unquenchable thirst.

In *Ayurveda,* the inner bark of the jambul tree is also used in the treatment of diabetes. The bark is dried and burnt, which produces an ash of white colour. This ash should be pestled in the mortar, strained and bottled. The diabetic patient should be given 65 mg. of this ash on an empty stomach with water in the morning and 135 mg. each time in the afternoon and in the evening, an hour after meals, if the specific gravity of the urine is 1.02 to 1.03. If the specific gravity ranges between 1.035 and 1.055, the ash should be given thrice daily in the quantity of about 2 gm. at a time.[1]

### Polyuria

The powder of the seeds is valuable in polyuria or production of excess urine. It should be taken in dose of 1 gm. in the morning and evening.

### Diarrhoea and Dysentery

Powder of the seed is an effective remedy for diarrhoea and dysentery. About 5 to 10 gm. of this powder should be taken with butter-milk in these conditions. An infusion of the tender leaves, which contain a high concentration of gallic and tannic acid is also given as a medicine in diarrhoea and dysentery. This infusion, prepared from 30 or 60 gm. of leaves, should be given twice or thrice daily. A decoction of the bark taken with honey is also an useful medicine for chronic diarrhoea and dysentery.[2]

### Piles

The jambul fruit is an effective food remedy for bleeding piles. The fruit should be taken with salt every morning for two or three months in its season. The use of the fruit in this manner in every season will effect radical cure and save the user from bleeding piles for entire life. Fresh jambul fruit taken with honey is also an effective medicine for bleeding piles.

### Liver Disorders

Natural acids in the jambul fruit play an important role in the secretion of digestive enzymes and stimulate the liver functions. Charaka, the well-known physician of the ancient India, used this fruit in the treatment of enlargement of the liver.

### Female sterility

An infusion of the fresh tender leaves of jambul fruit, taken with honey or butter-milk, is an effective remedy for sterility and

1. Kvj. Ganpati Singh Verma, *Miracles of Indian Herbs,* p. 61, Rasayan Pharmacy, 1982.

2. Dr. Aman, *Medicinal Secrets of Your Food,* pp. 223-224, Indo-American Hospital, Mysore, 1985.

miscarriage due to overian or endometrium functional disorder. The leaves presumably stimulate the secretion of progrestrone hormone and help absorption of vitamin E.

**Precautions**

The jambul fruit should not be consumed in excess. Its excessive use is bad for throat and chest. It may cause cough and accumulation of sputum in the lungs.

# *Lemon*

Botanical Name : *Citrus limon*
Indian Names : *Bara nimbu, Pahari nimbu*

**Description**

The lemon is an important fruit of citrus group. It ranks high as a health food. It is sometimes mistaken for the lime, but the lime is a smaller species and the lemon forms a bigger variety, with a rough, thin and loose rind.

Lemon is oval in shape and light yellow in colour with thick, rough skin. When ripe it has pale yellow pulp, abundant juice and a small number of seeds.

**Origin and Distribution**

The lemon is indigenous to the north-west regions of India, ascending to an altitude of 4,000 ft. It has been cultivated in south-east Asia from ancient times. It reached Europe in the 12th and 13th centuries. It is now widely grown in all tropical and subtropical countries, notably in the United States, Spain, Portugal, France, West Indies and New South Wales. In India, lemon is cultivated in home gardens and small-sized orchards in parts of Uttar Pradesh, Bombay, Madras and Mysore.

**Food Value**

The lemon is rich in many food ingredients, particularly citric acid. Different varieties contain this acid in different proportions ranging from 3.71 to 8.40 per cent. It is mainly due to its citric acid and Vitamin C contents that the lemon is widely used in medicine. It is valued for its juice which is mostly used as an accessory food. It increases the flavour and improves the taste of various dishes. It is often used in the preparation of salads and prevents and disclouration of sliced bananas and apple. It is widely used in the preparation of lemonades, squashes, jams, jellies and marmalades. The lemon juice has a good keeping quality and it can be preserved for a long time with certain precautions.

**Lemon\***

| Food Value | | Minerals and Vitamins | |
|---|---|---|---|
| Moisture | 85.0% | Calcium | 70 mg |
| Protein | 1.0% | Phosphorus | 10 mg |
| Fat | 0.9% | Iron | 2.3 mg |
| Minerals | 0.3% | Vitamin C | 39 mg |
| Fibre | 1.7% | Small amount of | |
| Carbohydrates | 11.1% | Vitamin B Complex | |
| | 100% | | |

\*Value per 100 gms edible portion          **Calorific Value - 57**

## Natural Benefits and Curative Properties

The various parts of the lemon used for medicinal purposes are rind of the ripe fruit, essential oil of the rind and expressed juice of the ripe fruit. A pale yellow volatile oil is derived either through distillation or by squeezing out from fresh outer part of the paricarp of the fruit. Though the oil is bitter yet it is highly valued in medicine as a flavouring agent, carminative that relives flatulence for treating gastric discomfort and stomachic that improves appetite. Rind is also both stomachic and carminative. Lemon juice, the expressed and strained juice of the ripe fruit, is valuable as antiscorbutic and refrigerant. It destroys the toxins in the body. This detoxifying property arises from its high potassium content. The germs of diptheria, typhoid and other deadly diseases are destroyed by its use. The juice also encourages bile secretion and is valuable in jaundice and gravels—a condition of small stone in urinary tract. The bark of the lemon tree is used as febrifuge which prevents fever and seeds as a vermifuge which expels worms from intestine.

### Scurvy

The lemon is chiefly valued for its vitamin C content. Its juice contains more vitamin than the whole fruit, being about 60 mg. per 100 gram. The juice also contains appreciable quantity

of vitamin **B**. This makes it antiscorbutic or an excel[...]
medicine for the prevention and treatment of scurvy. A[...]
of one part of lemon juice, three parts of water and a[...]
quantity of sugar or honey should be taken in this co[...]

## Oral Diseases

Due to its high content of vitamin C, lemon strengthens the gums and teeth. It is also very effective for preventing and curing acute inflammations of the gum margins, pyorrhoea, dental caries and other oral diseases.

## Throat Disorders

Lemon is highly beneficial in the treatment of throat disorders such as catarrh, choking sensation and itching sensitivities. A ripe unpeeled lemon should be roasted slowly until it begins to crack open. Then one teaspoonful of the juice with a little honey should be taken once every hour, or the same juice of the roasted lemon in a glass of boiled water should be taken flavoured with honey. It should be sipped slowly.

## Burning Soles and Heels

Sliced lemon should be rubbed over the entire burning soles and heals of feet. A great deal of toxin elimination takes place through the pores of the feet. Lemon application promotes such elimination and keep the feet free from pain and distress.

## Digestive Problems

A ripe lemon is a good appetiser. The lemon juice stimulates the flow of saliva and gastric juice and is regarded as an excellent digestive agent. It destroys intestinal worms and eliminates the gases formed in the digestive tract. It is highly beneficial in the treatment of several digestive problems like dyspepsia, constipation and biliousness. Heartburn is easily relieved by taking the juice of half a lemon in a little water.

## Fevers

Lemon juice makes an effective thirst-quenching drink in pox, measles, scarlet and other fevers which are attendent with extreme thirst and a very hot and dry skin. About 15 to 25 gm. of lemon juice should be taken in these conditions.

## Haemorrhage

Lemon is effective in the haemorrhage or bleeding of lungs, stomach, intestines, uterus, kidneys and other internal organs.

.n these cases, lemon juice should be taken with water several tiems a day.[1]

**Enlargement of Spleen**

Lemons are valuable in the case of enlargement of spleen. Two lemons, cut up into halves and slightly heated after adding a little salt, have proved beneficial in this condition.

**Rheumatic Affections**

Though the lemon juice is sour in taste, its reaction in the body is alkaline and as such it is valuable in the treatment of rheumatic affections such as gout, rheumatism, sciatica, lumbago, pain in hip joints which result from too much acid in the body. A sufficient intake of lemon juice prevents the deposit of uric acid in the tissues and thus reduces the possibility of an attack of gout.

**Obesity**

An exclusive lemon juice is an effective remedy for obesity. On the first day the patient should be given nothing but plenty of water. On the second day juice of three lemons mixed with equal amount of water should be given. One lemon should be subsequently increased each day until the juice of 12 lemons is consumed per day. Then the number of lemons should be decreased in the same order until three lemons are taken in a day. The patient may feel weak and hungry on first two days, but afterwards the condition will stabilise by itself.

**Cold**

London's first influenza epidemic in November 1931 was cured, not by doctors, but by lemon. Some one has appropriately said, "A lemon a day keeps a cold away." For a bad cold, the juice of two lemons in half-a-litre of boiling water, sweetened with honey, taken at bed time, is a very effective remedy.[2]

**Circulatory Disorders**

The lemon is a rich source of vitamin P and it contains 1.75 mg. of this vitamin per 100 gm. It is found both in the juice and peel of the fruit. This vitamin is essential for controlling haemorrhage in a variety of conditions and for preventing

---

1. K.R. Mukherjee, *Protective Foods in Health and Disease*, p. 97, Prakritick Chikitsalaya, Calcutta, Fourth Edition, 1983.

2. Dr. S.J. Singh, *Food Remedies*, p. 116, Nature Cure Council of Medical Research, Lucknow, 1982.

capillary fragility. It is, therefore, regarded as a valuable medicine in high blood pressure and arterio-sclerosi strengthens the entire arterial system and consequently, value in many circulatory disorders and heart weakness.

Lemon peel is equally effective in these disorders. Shredded lemon peel may be added to soups and stews, or sprinkled over salad. To make a medicine, the peel of one or two lemons may be cut finely and keep in warm water for about 12 hours. A teaspoonful may be taken every three hours, or immediately before or after a meal.

## Cholera

Lemon has been provided by nature with wonderful anticholera properties. Lemon juice can kill cholera bacilli within a very short time. It is also a very effective and reliable preventive food item against cholera during the epidemic. For this purpose, it can be taken in the form of sweetened or salted beverages. Taking of lemon with food as a daily routine also saves from cholera.

## Foot Relaxation

Those who have to walk long distances will derine comfort by often soaking their feet in hot water and then a thorough rubbing of the feet with lemon juice. The benefit here is in the contrasting actions of the hot water which opens the pores and the lemon juice which presents a cooling, astringent action. This treatment is also said to promote healthy sleep, owing to its relaxing action on the foot nerves.[3]

## Corn

Lemon is valuable in corns. A fresh slice of lemon should be tied over the painful area at night and it should be allowed to remain there whole night.

## Beauty Aid

Lemon is regarded as a youth restorative. It helps create youthful health. To help cleanse blemished skin, the area should be rubbed with a fresh piece of lemon. The juice should be soaked into the skin, allowing it to remain overnight. Strained fresh lemon juice mixed with cool water should be used to wash

3. Eric F.W. Powell, *Health from the Kitchen*, p. 16, Health Science Press, England, 1973.

the hair to add to their brightness. Dry or scaly skin should be rubbed with the peel of a lemon. It will restore the skin to softness. Rough elbows can be soften by rubbing the area with the cut side of a lemon.[4]

# *Lime*

Botanical Name : *Citrus aurantifolia*
Indian Name : *Niboo*

### Description

The lime is an imporant fruit of citrus group. It is very popular all through the tropics and is used as a necessary adjunct in everyday meal. It is regarded as a health-building food of great value. Limes are generally mistaken for lemons, but they represent two varieties of the same genus. The lime is smaller in size than the lemon, with a thin smooth skin. It has sweet smell and contains less juice than the lemon. The lime grows on a small, multi-branched tree upto 5 m. in height, with spiny branches, small green leaves and white and strongly scented flowers.

There are many varieties of limes, differing in size, colour and shape. They are, however, classified into two main groups, namely, the sweet and the acid limes. The sweet limes contain a higher proportion of sugar but they have an insipid taste and are not considered to be of high nutritive value. They are, therefore, not grown on any great scale. Acid or sour limes, on the other hand, are extensively cultivated as their importance as food and medicine has been recognised for centuries. The two most popularly known varieties are *Pati* and *Kagzi niboo*.

### Origin and Distribution

The lime is believed to have originated in India, where it has been grown since remote times. Arab traders are believed to have taken it to Eastern Mediterranean and Western countries in about 1000 AD. The Spaniards took it to the New World early in

4. Carlson Wade, *Health Secrets from the Orient,* p.133, Allied Publishers Pvt. Ltd., Bombay.

their colonization. It has since spread throughout the tropics, where it is the most commonly cultivated species of the acid citrus.

**Food Value**

Acid limes are excellent source of free citric acid, natural sugar, vitamin C, calcium and phosphorus. It contains by far more vitamin C than the lemon. It is generally used for its juice which is taken in various ways. The best way to use it is to take with water. The lime juice forms an indispensable ingredient of salads. In fruit salads, it helps to retain the normal colour of fruits and imparts tart flavour. It is often mixed with cooked pulses, soups, sauces and gravies to make them more tasty and palatable.

**Lime\***

| Food Value | | Minerals and Vitamins | |
|---|---|---|---|
| Moisture | 84.6% | Calcium | 90 mg |
| Protein | 1.5% | Phosphorus | 20 mg |
| Fat | 1.0% | Iron | 0.3 mg |
| Minerals | 0.7% | Vitamin C | 63 mg |
| Fibre | 1.3% | Small amount of | |
| Carbohydrates | 10.9% | Vitamin B Complex | |
| | 100% | | |

\*Value per 100 gms edible portions          **Calorific Value -59**

## Natural Benefits and Curative Properties

The juice of fresh limes is being used in medicine from ancient times in India. In *Vadas*, lime has been mentioned as a sacred fruit. Cutting limes after reciting certain *Mantras* is considered an effective method for driving away the evil spirits. Charaka and Sharangdhara, the two famous physicians of ancient India, have mentioned about the therapeutic value of lime in various diseases of bones and joints. The vitamin C content in lime increases the body's resistance to disease, aids the healing of wounds and prevents damage to the eyes. Vitamin C is also helpful in maintaining the health of the teeth and other bones of the body. It prevents decay and loosening of the teeth, dental caries, toothache, bleeding of the gums and fragility of bones.

The rind of the fruit also has medicinal properties. It

contains a volatile oil which is used in medicine for improving digestion and removing wind.

## Scurvy

As a rich source of vitamin C, the lime has been regarded as a food of exceptional therapeutic value. It has saved the lives of innumerable crews of ocean-going vessels from scurvy. The Boards of Trade regulations have made it compulsory for the crew to have a supply of lime juice when vegetables are not available.

## Digestive Disorders

Lime is considered highly beneficial in the treatment of digestive disorders. A teaspoonful of fresh lime-juice should be mixed with equal quantity of honey. It should be licked to stop bilious vomiting, indigestion, burning in the chest due to high acidity in the stomach and excessive accumulation of saliva in the mouth.

A teaspoonful of lime juice mixed with water and a pinch of sodabicarb makes an excellent remedy for reducing the acidity in the stomach. It also acts as a powerful carminative in case of indigestion. It produces a marked sedative effect in the stomach due to release of carbonic acid gas.[1]

## Constipation

The lime juice is of great value in constipation, when it is taken as the first thing in the morning in a glass of warm water. In chronic cases, it helps remove the disorder by promoting biliary secretion from liver.

## Peptic Ulcers

The citric acid in limes has an alkaline reaction in the system. This acid together with the mineral salts present in the juice, helps the digestion by assisting in the absorption of fats and alcohol and by neutralising excessive bile produced by the liver. The juice counteracts the effects of greasy food and reduces gastric acidity. It is, therefore, specially valuable in the treatment of peptic ulcers.[2]

---

1. Dr. Aman, *Medicinal Secrets of Your Food,* pp. 227-228, Indo-American Hospital, Mysore, 1985.

2. Henlen Jeans, *About Tropical Fruits,* p. 40, Thorsons Publishers Ltd.,London, 1972.

## Common Cold

Lime is ideal in all types of fevers and cold if taken well-diluted. Vitamin C rich lime juice increases resistance, reduces toxicity and cuts down the course of the illness. Unless one is specially allergic to citrus fruits, one should not avoid lime in cold. A glass of diluted lime juice prepared in warm water, to which a teaspoonful of honey is added, is an ideal remedy for cold and dry cough.

## Tonsillitis

Lime has proved effective in the treatment of acute tonsillitis. A fresh lime squeezed in a glass of warm water, with four teaspoonful of honey and a quarter teaspoonful of common salt, should be sipped slowly in such cases.

## Gums

Lime is valuable in swollen gums. A glass of diluted fresh lime juice mixed with a pinch of rock salt should be taken in this condition. The squeezed lime rind should also be rubbed over the gums, before throwing it away.

## Gout

The fruit has been used as a remedy in gout and arthritis since long. Vitamin C is known to prevent and cure sore joints by strengthening the connective tissues of the body. The citric acid found in the lime is a solvent of the uric acid which is the primary cause of gout and other diseases of this nature.

## Eye Disorders

Lime juice is valuable in eye disorders. Few drops of warm lime-juice diluted with water should be instilled in the eyes in case of conjunctivitis. Its regular use with pure rose water in the ratio of 1:4 is helpful in preventing old-age cataract.[3]

## Bleeding Piles

A small lime should be slit into two and sprinkled with rock salt powder inside. The lime is then tucked inside the mouth and the juice slowly taken in. Lime juice, with its antihaemorrhagic properties and rock salt rich in magnesium sulphate, checks bleeding, help good bowel movement and gradually shrink the pile masses.

---

3. Dr. Aman, *Medicinal Secrets of Your Food,* p. 229, Indo-American Hospital, Mysore, 1985.

## Cystitis

Lime has proved valuable in cystitis—i.e.,inflammation of urirnary bladder. A teaspoonful of lime juice should be put in 180 gm. of boiling water. It should then be allowed to cool and 60 gm. of this water should be given every two hours in this condition. It gives relief to burning sensation and also stops bleeding in cystitis.

## Scorpion Sting

When externally applied, fresh lime is highly beneficial in the treatment of scorpion sting. A crystal of potassium permanganate should be put over it. It will have effect in ten minutes.

## Obesity

The lime juice is also excellent for weight reduction. It has a sedative effect on the nerves. Fresh juice of a lime mixed in a glassful of water and sweetened with honey should be taken every morning on empty stomach in case of obesity. It will reduce the weight in two to three months time. One should however, take low calorie diet to get the desired result.

## Beauty Aid

Lime can be used as a beauty aid. A fresh lime may be squeezed in a fully-boiled glassful of whole milk. A teaspoonful of glycerine may be added to it. It should be left for half an hour and then applied on the face, hands and feet before retiring at night. This application every night will help one to look young and beautiful. The application can also cure pimple, cracked soles and plams, dryness of the face and hand and protect the face from hot and cold winds and sun-burn. Massaging few drops of lime juice with *amla* juice every night before going to bed, stops falling of hair, lengthens them and prevents them from premature greying. It also cures dandruff.

## Precaution

Limes should not be used in excess. The alkaline salts of the lime juice neutralise the free uric acid and precipitate it. It has, therefore, been found that its excessive use may cause the formation of renal calculi.

Excessive sucking of fresh lime is also bad for teeth as the acid damages the delicate enamel of the teeth and makes them sensitive. Its excessive use weakens digestion and improverishes the blood.

# Mango

Botanical Name : *Mangifera indica*
Indian Name : *Aam*

## Description

The mango enjoys a unique status among the fruits. It is the most popular fruit of the tropics and is called 'The King of Asiatic fruits'. It is regarded as a valuable item of diet and a household remedy. The mango is fleshy drupe, variable in size and shape, with varying mixtures of green, yellow and red colour. Inside the fruit is stony endocarp, variable in size. Mango grows on a large, erect, branched, evergreen tree. The leaves, when fully grown, are stiff, pointed and deep glossy green. These are used in ceremonial decorations. The dry twigs are used to light sacred fires. The worst type of mangoes are very fibrous with turpentine flavour, but the best are juicy, sweet, with very little fibre and a deliciously piquant flavour.

## Origin and Distribution

The mango is indigenous to India. It has been cultivated here for over 4000 years. In *Vedas,* mango is praised as a heavenly fruit. In Hindu mythology; it is believed that when Lord Shiva and Parvati came from Himalayas, they missed this heavenly fruit. Parvati who was very fond of mango, requested her husband to create mango tree by his Divine Power. Lord Shiva fulfilled her desire and mango appeared in India.

Alexander and his armymen were the first Europeans who saw mango fruit in India in 327 BC. It was probably taken to Malaya and neighbouring East Asian countries by Indians in the fifth century BC and to the East African coast by Persians about 10th century AD.

Besides India, the fruit is now widely grown in China, Pakistan, Bangladesh, Philippines, Haiti, Mexico and Brazil. Numerous varieties are cultivated. In India alone, there are over 500 varieties, but only about 35 varieties are extensively cultivated.

## Food Value

The mango is used as food in all stages of its development. Green or unripe mango contains a large portion of starch which

63

gradually changes into glucose, sucrose and maltose as the fruit begins to ripe. It disappears completely when the fruit is fully ripe. Green mango is a rich source of pectin which gradually diminishes after the formation of the stone. Unripe mango is sour in taste because of the presence of oxalic, citric, malic and succinic acids.

**Mango\***

| Food Value | | Minerals and Vitamins | |
|---|---|---|---|
| Moisture | 81.0% | Calcium | 14 mg |
| Protein | 0.6% | Phosphorus | 16 mg |
| Fat | 0.4% | Iron | 1.3 mg |
| Minerals | 0.4% | Vitamin C | 16.0% |
| Fibre | 0.7% | Small amount of | |
| Carbohydrates | 16.9% | Vitamin B Complex | |
| | 100% | | |

\*Value per 100 gms edible portion      **Calorific Value -74**

The raw mango is a valuable source of vitamin C. It contains more vitamin C than half-ripe or fully ripe mangoes, It is also a good source of vitamin $B_1$ and $B_2$ and contains sufficient quantity of niacin. These vitamins differ in concentration in various varieties during the stages of maturity and environmental conditions.

The ripe fruit is very wholesome and nourishing. The chief food ingredient of mango is sugar. The acids contained in the fruit are tartaric acid and malic acid, besides a trace of citric acid. These acids are utilised by the body and they help to maintain the alkali reserve of the body.

**Natural Benefits and Curative Properties**

The mango is well-known for its medicinal properties both in unripe and ripe states. The unripe fruit is acidic, astringent and antiscorbutic. The skin of the unripe fruit is astringent and stimulant tonic. The bark is also astringent and has a marked action on mucous membranes.[1] Mango pickles preserved in oil and salted solution is used throughout India. However, these pickles, if extremely sour, spicy and oily, are not good for health and should be specially avoided by those suffering from arthritis,

---

1. J.F. Dartur, *Medicinal Plants of India & Pakistan,* p. 106, D.B. Taraporevala Sons & Co. (P) Ltd., Bombay, 1985.

rheumatism, sinusitis, sore throat and hyperacidity.

The ripe mango is antiscorbutic, diuretic, laxative, invigorating, fattening and astringent. It tones up the heart muscle, improves complexion and stimulates appetite. It increases the seven body nutrients, called 'dhatus' in *Ayurveda*. They are food juice, blood, flesh, fat, bone marrow and semen. The fruit is beneficial in liver disorders, loss of weight and other physical disturbances.

## Unripe Mango
## Heat Stroke

The unripe mango protects men from the adverse effects of hot, scorching winds. A drink, prepared from the unripe mango by cooking it in hot ashes and mixing the pith with sugar and water, is an effective remedy for heat exhaustion and heat stroke. Eating raw mango with salt quenches thirst and prevents the excessive loss of sodium choloride and iron during summer due to excessive sweating.

**Gastro-Intestinal Disorders :** Unripe green mangoes are beneficial in the treatment of gastro-intestinal disorders. Eating one or two small tender mangoes in which the seed is not fully formed with salt and honey is found to be very effective medicine for summer diarrhoea, dysentery, piles, morning sickness, chronic dyspepsia, indigestion and constipation.[2]

### Bilious Disorders

Unripe mangoes are an excellent fruit remedy for bilious disorders. The acids contained in the green mango increase the secretion of bile and act as intestinal antiseptic. Therefore, eating green mango daily with honey and pepper cures biliousness, food putrefaction i.e. when proteins are decomposed by bacteria; urticaria and jaundice. It tones up the liver and keeps it healthy.[3]

### Blood Disorders

The green mango is valuable in blood disorders because of its high vitamin C content. It increases the elasticity of the blood vessels and helps the formation of new blood cells. It aids the

---

2. Hakeem Rasool Sahib, *Jiryan-Ka-illaj,* (Urdu Mss.) 289, Mandi Mohalla, Mysore, 1930.

3. Hakeem Mahboob Ali Khan Bakshi, *Amm-say-Bimarioon-ka Illaj,* (Urdu Mss.) Mandi Mohalla, Mysore, 1959.

tion of food-iron and prevents bleeding tendencies. It
ses body resistance against tuberculosis, anemia, cholera
, sentery.

## Scurvy

The *amchur*, a popular article of diet in Indian houses,
consists of green mangoes skinned, stoned, cut into pieces and
dried in the sun. 15 gm. of it is believed to be equivalent to 30 gm.
of good lime on account of its citric content. It is valuable in the
treatment of scurvy.[4]

## Ripe Mango
## Eye Disorders

Ripe mangoes are highly beneficial in the treatment of night
blindness in which one cannot see properly in dim light. This
disease is caused by vitamin A deficiency. It is very common
among children who are victim of malnutrition due to poverty.
Liberal use of mangoes during the season will be very effective in
such conditions. It will also prevent many other eye diseases
which may ultimately cause total blindness. Eating mangoes
liberally will also prevent development of refractive errors,
dryness of the eyes, softening of the cornea, itching and burning
in the eyes.[5]

## Infections

All bacterial invasions are due to poor epithelium the tissue
that covers the external surface fo the body. Liberal use of
mangoes during the season contributes towards formation of
healthy epithelium, thereby preventing frequent attacks of
common infections such as colds rhinitis and sinusitis. This is
attributable to high concentration of vitamin A in mangoes.

## Loss of Weight

The mango-milk cure is an ideal treatment for loss of weight.
For this mode of treatment, ripe and sweet mangoes should
always be selected. They should be taken thrice a day—morning,
noon and evening. The mangoes should be taken first and then
followed by milk. The mango is rich in sugar but deficient in
protein. On the other hand, milk is rich in protein but deficient

---

4. Dr. S.J. Singh, *Food Remedies,* p. 128, Nature Cure Council of
Medical Research, Lucknow, 1982.

5. Dr. Aman, *Medicinal Secrets of Your Food,* p. 256, Indo-American
Hospital, Mysore, 1985.

in sugar. The deficiency of the one is made up by the other. Mango thus combines very well with milk and exclusive mango-milk diet taken for at least one month, will lead to improvement in health, vigour and gain in weight. The quantity of milk and of the mangoes to be consumed in this mode of treatment should be carefully regulated according to the condition of the patient. For rapid gain in weight, about 4 to 5 litres of milk should be consumed with 3 to 4 kg. of mangoes.

**Diabetes**

The tender leaves of the mango tree are considered useful in diabetes. An infusion is prepared from fresh leaves by soaking them overnight in water and squeezing them well in water before filtering it in the morning. This infused water should be taken every morning to control early diabetes. As an alternative to infusion. leaves can be dried in the shade, powdered and preserved. Half a teaspoonful of this powder should be taken twice a day, in the morning and evening.

**Diarrhoea**

The mango seeds are valuable in diarrhoea. The seeds should be collected during the mango season, dried in the shade and powdered and stored for use as medicine. It should be given in doses of about one and a half gram to two grams with or without honey. Juice of fresh flowers when taken with one or two teaspoonful of curds, is also valuable in diarrhoea.

**Female Disorders**

Mango seeds are considered useful in certain disorders connected with women's reproductive organs. According to Dr. Aman, 'A teaspoonful of the paste of the decorticated kernel of mango is applied inside the vagina to cure lucorrhoea, vaginitis, and relaxed walls due to multiple pregnancies. Its use half an hour before conjugal union gives a virgin feeling and acts as a safe contraceptive. This has been tried many times with gratifying results.[6]

Juice of the fresh mango bark is also valuable in heavy bleeding during menstruation, i.e. menorrhagia, leucorrhoea, mucus and pus discharges from the uterus and bleeding or haemorrhage from uterus. The juice is given with the addition

---

6. Dr. Aman, *Clinical Observation of Mango Kernal on the Mortality of Sperms and its Spermicidal Action*, p. 120, 1962-67.

of white of an egg or some mucilage—a kind of vegetable glue obtained from plant and a little opium in these diseases. In the alternative, a mixture of 10 ml. of a fluid extract of the bark and 120 ml. of water is given in doses of a teaspoonful every hour or two.

**Throat Disorders**

The mango bark is very efficacious in the treatment of diphtheria and other throat diseases. Its fluid is locally applied and also used as a gargle. The gargle is prepared by mixing 10 ml. of the fluid extract with 125 ml. of water.

**Scorpion Bites**

The juice which oozes out at the time of plucking the fruit from the tree gives immediate relief to pain when applied to a scorpion bite or the sting of a bee. The juice can be collected and kept in a bottle.

**Precautions**

Unripe mangoes should not be eaten in excess. Their excessive intake may cause throat irritation, indigestion, dysentery and abdominal colic. One should, therefore, not consume more than one or two green mangoes daily. Water should not be drunk immediately after eating the green mango because it coagulates the sap and makes it more irritant. Sap or milky juice which comes out on breaking the stalk of the green mango is irritant and astringent. Eating green mangoes without draining the sap may cause mouth, throat and gastro intestinal irritations. The sap should, therefore be fully squeezed out or the skin should be peeled before using raw mango.

Excessive use of mangoes produce ailments like constipation, eye affections, blood impurities and seasonal fever. Children who use the fruit in excess generally suffer from skin disease in its season.

# *Orange*

Botanical Name : *Citrus aurantium*
Indian Name : *Santrā*

**Description**

The orange is one of the finest gifts of nature. It is the most popular wide-spread of the citrus fruits. It is a very delicious and nourishing fruit which is upto 12 cm. in diameter, though most common ones are only 6 to 8 cm. in diameter. The fruit grows on a spreading evergreen tree, upto 12 m. tall, with dark green leaves and fragrant flowers.

There are many varieties of oranges. The more important ones are loose-skinned orange, tight-skinned orange and sour-orange. The loose-skinned orange is very popular in India and the tight-skinned one is very popular in Europe.

**Origin and Distribution**

The orange is a native of southern China. It is believed to have been introduced into south India from where it was taken to the western world by Vasco da Gama in 1498. However, it did not spread in India and the present cultivated varieties were introduced from abroad. It is extensively cultivated in the U.S.A., Spain, Brazil, China, Japan, Palestine, Italy, South Africa, Egypt and Mexico. In India, the loose-skinned orange grows widely in Nagpur and Pune in Maharashtra state, Assam and Coorg.

**Food Value**

The orange is a rich source of protective food ingredients lik vitamins A, B, C and calcium and its health-promotin properties emanate from this fact. It is superior to almost an) other fruit as a source of calcium. The orange also contains sodium, potassium, magnesium, copper, sulphur and chlorine.

| Orange* | | | |
|---|---|---|---|
| **Food Value** | | **Minerals and Vitamins** | |
| Moisture | 87.6% | Calcium | 26 mg |
| Protein | 0.7% | Phosphates | 20 mg |
| Fat | 0.2% | Iron | 0.3 mg |
| Minerals | 0.3% | Vitamin C | 30 mg |
| Fibre | 0.3% | Small amounts of | |
| Carbohydrates | 10.9% | Vitamin B Complex | |
| | 100% | | |
| *Values per 100 gms edible portions | | **Calorific Value -59** | |

Its vatamin C content helps the body tissues to use the calcium contained in the food.

69

## Natural Benefits and Curative Properties

The orange is a predigested food as the starch of the orange is converted into readily assimilable sugar by the rays of the sun. It is thus readily absorbed in the blood. It produces heat and energy in the body immediately after its use.

The regular use of orange prevents frequent attacks of common cold, influenza and bleeding tendencies. It keeps one healthy and strong and contribute towards longevity. Orange juice, among all the fruit juices, is more suitable for all ages and can be given with advantage in all kinds of diseases.

### Fevers

Orange is an excellent food in all types of fever when the digestive power of the body is seriously hampered. The fever patient suffer from blood poisoning called toxaemia and the lack of saliva coats his tongue and often destroys his thirst for water as well as his desire for food. The agreeable flavour of orange juice helps greatly in overcoming these drawbacks. Orange juice is the most ideal liquid food in fevers like typhoid, tuberculosis and measles. It gives energy, increases urinary output and promotes body resistance against infections, thereby, hastening recovery.

### Dyspepsia

The orange is an effective food remedy in chronic dyspepsia. It gives rest to the digestive organs and supplies nutrition in a most easily assimilable form. It also stimulates the flow of digestive juices thereby improving digestion and increasing appetite. It creates suitable condition for the development of friendly bacteria in the intestines.

### Constipation

The orange is beneficial in the treatment of constipation. Taking one or two oranges at bedtime and again on rising in the morning is an excellent way of stimulating bowel action. The general stimulating influence of orange juice excites peristaltic activity and helps prevent the accumulation of food residue in the colon, which leads to putrefaction and auto-intoxication.[1]

---

1. Dr. S.J. Singh, *Food Remedies,* p. 152, Nature Cure Council of Medical Research, Lucknow, 1982.

## Diseases of Bone and Teeth

This fruit, being an excellent source of calcium and vitamin C, is valuable in the diseases of the bone and teeth. Disorders in the structure of the teeth usually result from shortage of vitamin C and calcium and these can be overcome by sufficient intake of orange. Dr. Harke, a Chicago physician, has claimed to have cured several patients of pyorrhoea and dental caries by giving them orange juice in large amounts.[2]

## Children's Ailments

Orange juice is considered an excellent food for infants who are not fed on breast milk. They should be given 15 ml. to 120 ml. of orange juice daily according to age. It prevents scurvy and rickets and helps growth. This juice can also be given with beneficial results to more grown up babies whose normal development is insatisfactory. They should be given 60 ml. to 120 ml. of orange juice daily.[3]

## Heart Disease

Orange juice, sweetened with honey, is highly beneficial in heart diseases. In cardiac conditions like coronary ischaemia and infarction, when only liquid food is advisable. The use of orange juice with honey is a very safe energy giving liquid food.[4]

## Difficult Expectorations

The use of orange juice mixed with a pinch of salt and a tablespoonful of honey is an effective food remedy for tuberculosis, asthma, common cold, bronchitis and other conditions of cough associated with difficult expectorations. Due to its saline action in the lungs, it eases expectorations and protects from secondary infection.

## Acne

The orange peel is valuable in the treatment of pimples and acne. The peel, pounded well with water on a piece of stone, should be applied to the affected areas. It is said to be more effective, if it is pounded with rain water.

2. J.B.S. Braverman, *Citrus Products*, p. 3, Interscience Publishers, Inc, New York, 1949.

3. K.R. Mukherjee, *Protective Foods in Health & Disease*, p. 136, Prakritick Chikitsalaya, Calcutta, 1983.

4. Dr. Aman, *Medicinal Secrets of Your Food*, p. 237, Indo-American Hospital, Mysore, 1985.

**Uses**

The orange is used in a variety of ways. It is usually taken as a dessert fruit. Large quantities of the fruit are used for making orange juice, which is canned. It is also made into squashes. Oranges are also used for marmalades and jams. Essential oil from the rind of the fruit is valued in perfumery.

# *Papaya*

Botanical Name : *Carica papaya*
Indian Name : *Papitā*

**Description**

The papaya has been regarded as one of the most valuable of tropical fruits. It is a large, fleshy, hollow berry upto 50-60 cm. in diameter and usually weighs from ½ kg. to 2 kg. It is cylindrical or pear-shaped. The central cavity is surrounded by hundreds of small seeds, though sometimes seedless varieties of the fruit are also found.

The fruit has a thin smooth skin. It is dark green in colour at first, but as the papaya ripens, it changes to bright yellowish or orange. Inside, the thick juicy flesh has a soft melting quality, and may be yellow or pink. It has a delicate aroma and delicious flavour.

**Origin and Distribution**

Papaya appears to have originated in southern Mexico and Costa Rica. It was taken by the Spaniards to Manila in the mid-16th century and gradually spread to all tropical and sub-tropical countries. It is now widely cultivated in India, China, Sri Lanka, Malaya, Mexico, Brazil, Peru, Venezuela, Central and South Africa, Philippines, Australia and on most of the Pacific islands.

**Food Value**

Papaya is regarded as a wholesome fruit. The daily requirements of some of the essential nutrients like proteins, mineral and vitamins can be met from this fruit. The vitamin C contents in papaya increases as the maturity progresses. Its carbohydrate

72

content is mainly of invert sugar which is a form of predigested food.

## Papaya*

| Food Value | | Minerals and Vitamins | |
| --- | --- | --- | --- |
| Moisture | 90.8% | Calcium | 17 mg |
| Protein | 0.6% | Phosphorus | 13 mg |
| Fat | 0.1% | Iron | 0.5 mg |
| Minerals | 0.5% | Vitamin C | 57 mg |
| Fibre | 0.8% | Small amount of | |
| Carbohydrates | 7.2% | Vitamin B Complex | |
| | 100% | | |
| *Values per 100 gms edible portion | | **Calorific Value - 32** | |

## Natural Benefits and Curative Properties

The papaya has remarkable medicinal virtues which were fully recognised even in ancient times. It is not only one of the most easily digested fruits, but it also aids the digestion of other foods. Ripe papaya is excellent tonic for growing children, for pregnant women and nursing mothers. It is an energy giving food.

### Digestive Aid

Modern scientific investigations into the properties of the papaya have confirmed many of the ancient beliefs in its virtues. The most important of these virtues is the discovery of a protein-digesting enzyme in the milky juice or latex, which is carried in a network of vessels throughout the plant. The enzyme is similar to pepsin in its digestive action and is reputed to be so powerful that it can digest 200 times its own weight in protein. Its effect is to assist the body's own enzymes in assimilating the maximum nutritional value from food to provide energy and body-building materials.[1]

### Intestinal Disorders

Papain in the raw papaya is highly beneficial in the deficiency of gastric juice, excess of unhealthy mucus in the stomach, in dyspepsia and intestinal irritation. The ripe fruit, if eaten regularly, corrects habitual constipation, bleeding piles and

---

1. Henlen Jeans, *About Tropical Fruits,* p. 49, Thorsons Publishers Ltd, London, 1972.

chronic diarrhoea. The juice of the papaya seeds is also useful in dyspepsia and bleeding piles.[2]

### Roundworms

The digestive enzyme papain in the milky juice of the unripe papaya is powerful anthelmintic for (i.e. which has the power to destroy) roundworms. A tablespoonful of the fresh juice and equal quantity of honey should be mixed with three to four tablespoonful of hot water and taken as a dose by an adult. This dose should be followed two hours later by a dose of 30 to 60 ml. of castor oil mixed in 250-375 ml. of luke warm milk. This treatment should be repeated for two days, if necessary. For children of 7 to 10 years, half the above doses should be given. For children under three years, a teaspoonful is sufficient.

Papaya seeds are also useful for this purpose, they are rich in a substance called caricin which is a very effective medicine for expelling roundworms. The alkaloid carpaine found in the leaves has also the power to destroy or expel intestinal worms. They are given with honey.

### Skin Disorders

The juice of the raw papaya, being an irritant, is useful in several skin disorders. It is applied with beneficial results to swellings to prevent pus formation or suppuration and to corns, warts, pimples, horn, an excrescence or an abnormal outgrowth of the skin and other skin diseases. The juice as a cosmetic, removes freckles or brown spots due to exposure to sunlight and makes the skin smooth and delicate. A paste of the papaya seeds is applied in skin diseases like ringworm.

### Menstrual Irregularities

The unripe papaya helps the contraction of the muscle fibres of the womb and is thus beneficial in securing proper menstrual flow. It is especially helpful in case of cessation of menstruation due to exposure to the cold or due to fright in young unmarried girls.

### Cirrhosis of the liver

Black seeds of papaya are highly beneficial in the treatment of cirrhosis of the liver caused by alcoholism, malnutrition etc. A tablespoonful of juice obtained by grinding the seeds, mixed

2. J.F. Dastur, *Medicinal Plants of India and Pakistan,* p. 47, D.B. Taraporevala & Sons & Co. (P) Ltd., Bombay, 1985.

with ten drops of fresh lime juice, should be given once or twice daily for about a month as a medicine for this disease.[3]

## Throat Disorders

Fresh juice of raw papaya mixed with honey can be applied with beneficial results over inflamed tonsils for diphtheria and other throat disorders. It dissolves the membrane and prevents infection from spreading.

## Spleen Enlargement

Ripe papaya is highly valuable in enlargement of the spleen. The fruit should be skinned, cut into pieces and immersed in vinegar for a week. About 20 grams of the fruit thus preserved should be consumed twice with meals in the treatment of this disease.[4] Slices of peeled raw fruit with cumin seeds and pepper can also be used once daily to cure enlargement of the spleen due to malaria.

## Uses

Papaya is used in a variety of ways. The ripe fresh fruits are eaten throughout the tropics for breakfast and dessert, and in fruit salads. They are used for making soft drinks, jams and ice-cream flavouring. They are also canned in syrup. Unripe fruits are generally taken as a vegetable.

Papain, prepared from the dried latex of immature fruits is used in meat-tenderizing preparation, manufacture of chewing-gum, in cosmetics and as a drug for digestive ailments.


# *Pomegranate*

Botanical Name : *Punica granatum*
Indian Name : *Anār*

## Description

The pomegranate is a very delicious and semi-seedy fruit. It has refreshing and soothing qualities and is more easy to digest

3. Dr. Aman, *Medicinal Secrets of Your Food*, p. 273, Indo-American Hospital, Mysore, 1985.

4. Hakeem H. Abdul Hameed Saheb, *The Complete Book of Home Remedies*, p. 116, Orient Paperbacks, Delhi, 1988.

than any other fruit. The fruit has been held in high esteem from time immemorial as a food and a medicine. It is symbolic of plenty and a basket of pomegranates was chosen as a symbol of the 18th International Horticultural Congress held in 1970. The pomegranate is a six-sided fruit of fairly large size, with tough leathery skin. It is divided inside into several cells containing numerous angular seeds. These seeds are surrounded by a succulent coating of pink or crimson colour with a delicious sub-acid flavour. The sweet ruby-pink and the sour varieties are most popular.

## Origin and Distribution

The pomegranate is a native of Iran and Afghanistan. It was grown in the hanging gardens of Babylon and was known in ancient Egypt. The pomegranate spread early round the Mediterranean and eastwards to India, China and Japan. In India, it is cultivated mostly around Pune, in Maharashtra and Dholka in Gujarat and to a limited extent in Uttar Pradesh.

**Pomegranate***

| Food Value | | Minerals and Vitamins | |
|---|---|---|---|
| Moisture | 78.0% | Calcium | 10 mg |
| Protein | 1.6% | Phosphorus | 70 mg |
| Fat | 0.1% | Iron | 0.3 mg |
| Minerals | 0.7% | Vitamin C | 16 mg |
| Fibre | 5.1% | Small amount of | |
| Carbohydrates | 14.5% | Vitamin B Complex | |
| | 100% | | |

*Values Per 100 gms edible portions · · · · · · · · **Calorific Value - 65**

## Curative and Medicinal Properties

The pomegranate has been regarded as a food medicine of great importance. All parts of the tree, the roots, the reddish brown bark, leaves, flowers, rind and seeds, have featured in medicine for thousands of years. The medical authorities of ancient India have described it as a light food and a tonic for the heart. The ancient medical writers of Arabia regarded it as a fruit which is good for the inflammation of the stomach and pain of the heart. The sweet varieties of the fruit are considered a good laxative, while those which are intermediate between sweet and sour are regarded as valuable in the stomach inflammations and heart pain.[1]

The juice from the fresh fruit is an excellent cooling beverage for alleviating thirst in cases of fevers and sickness. It acts on the liver, heart and kidneys and tones up their functions. It supplies the required minerals and helps the liver to preserve vitamin A from the food. It increases the body's resistance against infections, particularly tuberculosis.

## Digestive Disorders

Pomegranate juice is of great value in digestive disorders. It is an apetiser, a digestive food item and is useful for patients suffering from colitis and mucous. It binds the stools and tones up the intestines. A tablespoonful of the juice mixed with equal quantity of honey can be given with beneficial results in bilious vomiting i.e. bile containing fluid and nausea, burning in chest due to excessive secretion of bile, flatulent colic and morning sickness.

## Diarrhoea and Dysentery

The chief value of the pomegranate is its astringent properties which cause cells to shrink—and it is a valuable food medicine for diarrhoea and dysentery. If the patient develops weakness on account of profuse and continuous purging, he should be given repeatedly about 50 ml. of pomegranate juice to drink. This will control his diarrhoea. If the patient passes blood with stools, this will also stop by the use of fresh pomegranate juice. The flower buds are also astringent and are useful in chronic diarrhoea and dysentery, especially of children.[2]

## Intestinal Worms

The bark, both of the root and the stems of pomegranate tree, is well known for its anthelmintic properties of destroying parasitic worms. The root-bark is, however, preferred as it contains greater quantity of the alkaloid punicine than the stem-bark. This alkaloid is highly toxic to tapeworms. 90 to 180 ml. of the cold decoction of the bark, preferably fresh bark, should be given three times at an intervals of one hour to an adult. A purgative should be given after the last dose. The dose for children is 30 to

1. Helen Jeans, *About Tropical Fruits,* p. 68, Thorsons Publishers Ltd. London, 1972.

2. J.F. Dastur, *Medicinal Plants of India and Pakistan,* p. 139, D.B. Taraporevala Sons & Co. (P) Ltd., Bombay, 1985.

60 ml. The decoction is also used for expelling tapeworms.[3]

**Fevers**

The juice of the fruit with the addition of a little saffron is useful in fevers to allay thirst. A *sherbet* of the ripe fruit is beneficial in the treatment of typhus, gastric and asthmatic fevers. The root bark is also given as a febrifuge in—i.e. to prevent—fevers.[4]

**Anal Itching**

The skin of the pomegranate fruit is considered highly beneficial in the treatment of anal itching. This nasty discomfort may result from unhygienic habits or from worm infection. The skin of the fruit should be roasted till it is brittle and black. It is then powdered. The powder is mixed with a little vegetable oil and applied over the anus.

**Kidney and Bladder Stones**

The seeds of sour and sweet pomegranate are useful as a medicine. A tablespoonful of seeds, ground into a fine paste can be given along with a cupful of horse-gram soup to dissolve gravel in kidneys and bladder.

**Teeth and Gum Disorder**

Powder of the dry rind mixed with pepper and common salt is applied as a very good dentifrice—i.e. tooth paste or powder. Its regular application strengthens the gum, stops bleeding, prevents pyorrhoea, cleans the teeth and preserve them for a long time.

**Uses**

The pomegranate is used as a table-fruit. Its juice is regarded as a delicacy and is made into excellent *sherbet* and drunk with the addition of water and sugar. It is also used in preparing syrups, ice-creams, jellies and marmalades. The pomegranate has a very good keeping quality. It can be kept well for about six months in cold storage. Its thick rind protects its succulent seeds from much rough handling.

**Precautions**

The fruit should be eaten immediately after they are cut open

---

3. Ibid., PP. 139-140.
4. Dr. Aman, *Medicinal Secrets of Your Food*, p. 282; Indo-American Hospital, Mysore, 1985.

as the seeds lose their colour quickly. Pipes should not be swallowed while eating the fruit. This is said to have bad effect in the
intestines and may cause apendicitis.

# *Raisins*

Botanical Name : *Vitis vinifera*
Indian Name : *Munaqqā*

**Description**

The raisins are dried grapes. All grapes are, however, not
suitable for making raisins. The grapes, which are very sweet,
are only selected for drying. Raisins have high nourishing
qualities.

**Origin and Distribution**

Raisins have been used as food from very ancient times. They
had been known to the traders of the Mediterranean Coast even
in Greek and Roman ages. Raisins are produced in several parts
of the world, but the great bulk of world product comes from
Italy, France, Spain, Turkey, Iran, Afghanistan, Baluchistan,
California, Australia and South Africa.

**Food Value**

The raisins are esteemed for their rare food value. The table
below shows raisins are rich in carbohydrates, minerals and
vitamins. They form a very valuable food when taken with milk.
They supplement each other as the milk contains sufficient

## Raisins*

| Food Value | | Minerals and Vitamins | |
|---|---|---|---|
| Moisture | 20.2% | Calcium | 87 mg |
| Protein | 1.8% | Phosphorus | 80 mg |
| Fat | 0.3% | Iron | 7.7 mg |
| Minerals | 2.0% | Vitamin C | 1 mg |
| Fibre | 1.1% | Small amount of | |
| Carbohydrates | 74.6% | Vitamin B Complex | |
| | 100% | | |

*Values per 100 gms edible portions     **Calorific Value - 308** protein and the raisins, sugar. In same way they can be taken with advantage with nuts such as cashewnut, walnut and groundnut.

Raisins are extensively used in salads. They may be added to curries. They are also used in the bakery and confectionaries and widely used in the preparation of jams, jellies, cakes, puddings and pies.

## Natural Benefits and Curative Properties

The high food value of raisins arises chiefly from their sugar content. They contain eight times more sugar than grapes. The sugar contained in the raisins is of superior quality, like that of the grapes, as major portion of this sugar is formed by glucose and fruit sugar. As is well known, glucose produces quick heat and energy in the body. Raisins are thus an excellent food in all cases of debility and wasting diseases. They are also valuable during convalescence.

In Europe, persons suffering from various chronic ailments are taking recourse to an exclusive diet of raisins for some time. This forms a treatment by itself and is known as 'raisin cure'. It is believed that raisins, taken in this manner, for one month will bring about considerable improvement in health as a result of proper elimination.[1]

### Acidosis

Acidosis is a condition in which the acidity of body fluid is abnormally high. The raisins with their excess of alkalinity, are helpful in maintaining the acid balance of the body. Studies conducted by Saywell in the University of California have shown that the free use of raisins, say about 1.05 gm. daily, will greatly reduce the acidity of the urine. The urinary ammonia is also reduced. The organic acid of the raisins is completely oxidized. The free use of raisins is valuable in combating chronic acidosis which generally results from the excessive consumption of meat and cereals.[2]

### Constipation

Raisins are highly beneficial in the treatment of constipa-

1. K.R. Mukherjee, *Protective Foods in Health & Disease,* p. 175, Prakritick Chikitsalaya, Calcutta, 1983.

2. Dr. S.J. Singh, *Food Remedies,* p. 101, Nature Cure Council of Medical Research, Lucknow, 1982

tion They should be soaked in a glassful of drinking water for 24 to 48 hours This would swell them to the original size of the grapes. They should be eaten early in the morning, after discarding the stones. The water in which raisins are soaked should also be drunk This plan carried out every morning will bring excellent results in case of chronic constipation.

Raisins can be routinely given even to little infants as an extract in water to help regular bowel action. Six to ten raisins or more, depending on the child's age, can be soaked in boiling water and set aside for a while. When cool, the raisins should be thoroughly crushed to extract their juice into the water For small children, the liquid could be strained and given so that the skin of the raisins does not upset the stomach

### Anaemia

As a rich source of easily assimilable iron, raisins enrich blood They are thus useful in anaemia

### Under Weight

Raisins are a good food for those who wish to gain weight. They may be taken upto 1 Kg daily, 30 gm. or so at a time, in these cases

### Febrile Cases

An extract from raisins acts like a medicine in febrile cases i.e relating to fever This extract is prepared by soaking raisins in the water and then crushing them in the same water. They are then strained and skin is discarded. The raisin water thus prepared becomes a tonic A little lime juice added to the extract will enhance its taste and usefulness

### Sexual Debility

In *Ayurveda,* black raisins are used for restoration of sexual vigour. In such cases, they should be boiled with milk, after washing them thoroughly in tepid lukewarm water This will make them swollen and sweet. Eating of such raisins should be followed by the use of milk. Starting with 30 grams of raisins with 200 ml. of milk, three times daily. The quantity of raisins should be gradually increased to 50 grams each time

# Importance of Vegetables

'Vegetables' are important protective food and highly beneficial for the maintenance of health and prevention of disease. They contain valuable food ingredients which can be successfully utilised to build up and repair the body.

**Food Value**

Vegetables are valuable in maintaining alkaline reserve in the body. They are valued mainly for their high vitamin and mineral contents. Vitamins A, B and C are contained in vegetables in fair amounts. Faulty cooking and prolonged careless storage can, however, destroy these valuable elements.

There are different kinds of vegetables. They may be edible roots, stems, leaves, fruits and seeds. Each group contributes to diet in its own way. Fleshy roots are high in energy value and good sources of vitamin B group. Seeds are relatively high in carbohydrates and proteins. Leaves, steam and fruits are excellent sources of minerals, vitamins, water and roughage.

It is not the green vegetables only that are useful. Farinaceous vegetables consisting of starchy roots such as potatoes, sweet potatoes, the tubers and legumes are also valuable. They are excellent sources of carbohydrates and provide energy to the body.

**Natural Benefits**

To derive maximum benefits of their nutrients, vegetables should be consumed fresh as far as possible. Most vegetables are best consumed in their natural raw state in the form of salads. An important consideration in making salads is that the vegetables should be fresh, crisp and completely dry. If vegetables have to be cooked, it should be ensured that their nutritive value is preserved to the maximum extent possible. The following hints will be useful in achieving this :

i) The vegetables, after thorough wash, should be cut into as large pieces as possible.

ii) The cut pieces should be added to water which has been brought to boiling point and to which salt has been added. This is necessary to avoid loss of B-complex vitamins and vitamin C.

iii) Only bare minimum water necessary to cover vegetables should be used. Spinach and other tender greens need no water.

iv) Vegetables should not be exposed to atmospheric air They should be covered tightly while cooking

v) They should be cooked for as short a time as possible They should be cooked till they are just soft to the touch for easy mastication.

vi) They should be served hot.

To prevent loss of nutrients in vegetables, it would be advisable to steam or boil vegetables in their own juices on a slow fire and the water or cooking liquid should not be drained off. If the vegetables are boiled hard and for long time in a large quantity of water, they would lose their nutritive and medicinal values

No vegetable should be peeled unless it is so old that the peeling is tough and unpalatable. In most root vegetables, the largest amount of minerals is directly under the skin and these are lost if vegetables are peeled. Soaking of vegetables should also be avoided if taste and nutritive value are to be preserved.

Finally, vegetables should not be cooked in aluminium uten sils. Aluminium is a soft metal and is acted upon by both food acids and alkalis. There is scientific evidence to show that tiny particles of aluminium from foods cooked in such utensils enter the stomach and that the powerful astringent properties of aluminium injure the sensitive lining of the stomach, leading to gastric irritation, digestive and intestinal ailments.

An intake of about 280 grams of vegetables per day per person is considered essential for maintenance of good health. Of this, leafy vegetables should constitute 40 per cent, roots and tubers 30 per cent and the other vegetables like brinjals, ladies fingers the remaining 30 per cent.

### Vitamins

Many vegetables contain a substance known as carotene which is converted into vitamin A in the body. Vitamin A is essential for normal growth and vitality, for good eye-sight and healthy skin and for protection against diseases, especially of the respiratory tract. A deficiency of this vitamin can lead to eye infection, poor vision, night blindness, frequent colds, lack of appetite and skin disorders. Generally, deep green yellow and orange coloured vegetables such as green leafy vegetables, carrots, papaya tomatoes and yellow pumpkin are rich sources of carotene.

Several leafy vegetables like fenugreek leaves, turnip greens and beet green contain riboflavin, a member of the vitamin B-complex This vitamin is essential for growth and general health, of eyes, skin, nails and hair. A deficiency can lead to cracking of the angles of the mouth, premature wrinkles and eczema.

Vitamin C is contained in good amounts in several vegetables such as Indian gooseberry, bitter gourd, tomatoes and leafy vegetables like spinach, cabbage and drumstick leaves. Generally, fresh vegetables are better sources of vitamin C than dried, stale or withered ones. Vitamin C is essential for normal growth and maintenance of body tissues, especially those of the joints, bones, teeth and gums and for protection against infection. A deficiency of this vitamin can lead to scurvy, tooth decay, bleeding gums, anaemia and premature ageing.

### Minerals

The highly soluble minerals like calcium, phosphorus, iron, magnesium, copper, and potassium contained in the vegetables maintain the acid-base balance of the hydrogen concentration of the body tissues. They help the complete absorption of vitamins, proteins, fats and carbohydrates of the food. They also help the body to eliminate excess of liquid and salt. The diuretic action of vegetables like potato, beans, spinach, radish, turnip and brinjal are specially important in cases of oedema or swellings, kidney and heart conditions

Two important minerals, calcium and iron, found in vegetables are specially useful. Calcium is essential for strong bones and teeth. Iron is needed for blood formation. It is an essential constituent of haemoglobin, which helps to carry oxygen to the cells in the various parts of the body. Calcium and iron can be obtained in plenty from leafy vegetables like spinach and fenu greek leaves. Carrot, bitter gourd, onions and tomatoes are also fair sources of iron.

### Vegetable juices

The juices extracted from fresh raw vegetables are highly beneficial as they furnish all the cells and tissues of the body with the elements and the nutritional enzymes which they need. It is true that the body can derive these elements from whole vegeta bles. But the fresh juices can provide them in the manner in which they can be most easily digested and assimilated. A vitamin and mineral deficiency can thus be made much more quickly by drinking fresh juices than by eating raw vegetables

Practically all vegetables make good juices, but some bitter than others. Vegetable juices may be divided into three main types. These are (i) Juices from vegetable fruits, that is, tomatoes and cucumber (ii) Juices from green leafy vegetables such as cabbage, celery, lettuce, spinach and parsley and (iii) Juices from root vegetables like beetroot, carrot, onion, potato and radish

In most cases it is desirable to use juice individually and in no case more than three juices should be included in any one mix ture. The broad rules applicable to combination of vegetable juices are that juices from vegetable fruits may be combined with those of the green leafy vegetables but not juices of root vegetables. Juices of green leafy vegetables may be combined with those of the root vegetables.

Vegetable juices soothe jaded nerves and gently carry away toxic matter and accumulated waste products. They are best taken at least half an hour or more after meals. They should not be taken before meals or near the same time as fruit juices. Many common ailments respond favourably to raw vegetable juices.

### Curative Value

Vegetables contain various medicinal and therapeutic agents. There are a large array of laxatives, sedatives and soporif-ics or sleep inducing in the vegetable kingdom. Vegetables like onion, radish and celery exercise a tonic effect and are excellent for the nerves.

Certain vegetables are highly beneficial in the treatment of various diseases. Carrots are good for the blood. White crisp juicy stalks of celery serve a much better medicine in case of rheumatism or nervous dyspepsia than any nervine that relieves nurve disorder. A dish of spinach or dandelion will be beneficial in the treatment of kidney troubles. Lettuce can be used as a food remedy for insomnia. Onion can be used with advantage in the treatment of cough, cold, influenza, constipation, scurvy and hydrophobia. The leaves of fenugreek are highly valuable in the treatment of indigestion, flatulence and sluggish liver. Garlic can be beneficially used in heart diseases, hypertension, hypoglycemia, diabetes and even in fatal form of meningitis It has been effectively used in lowering blood cholesterol and preventing blood clotting.

## Gastro-Intestinal Disorders

Fibres in vegetables act as the mechanical intestinal expand ers draw more water and proteins in them and help easy expul sion of the waste in the form of stool. They prevent habitual constipation and keep the entire intestinal tract free from harm ful germs. Fibres in the form of cellulose help the elimination of cholesterol Beet root, cabbage, carrots, cucumbers, green peas and beans are especially valuable in this. They are useful in case of arteriosclerosis, high blood pressure and constipation. But when there is inflammation in this intenstines, vegetables having less cellulose content such as tomatoes, lettuce, potatoes and vegetable juices should be taken.

Pectin found in vegetables such as brinjal, radish, pumpkin and beet root absorb water, kill certain bacteria and toxins and eliminate them from the body. Garlic, onion, radish and mint contain pectin as well as anti-microbic qualities.

## Blood Disorder

Vegetables also supply trace elements which are necessary for the human organism. Iodine, for instance, is essential for thy roid hormone which regulates much physical and mental activi ties, cobalt for increasing the number of blood corpuscles, and zinc for proper growth.

# Amaranth

Botanical Name   *Amaranthus gangeticus*
Other English Name : *China spinach*
Indian Name : *Chaulai-ka-saag*

## Description

Amaranth is a popular green leafy vegetable grown all over India. It is usually a short-lived annual herb, with erect and often thick and fleshy stems and green leaves  There are about six different species of amaranth in cultivation

## Origin and Distribution

Most species of amaranth are believed to have originated in the Andran region of South America or Mexico. The various species are now widely distributed throughout most tropical areas—India, Malaysia, Indonesia, China, Taiwan, South Pacific, tropical Africa and the Caribbean  Amaranth is a warm-season crop and all species can be grown in the summer as well as the rainy season.

### Amaranth*

| Food Value | | Minerals and Vitamins | |
|---|---|---|---|
| Moisture | 85.7% | Calcium | 397 mg |
| Protein | 4.0% | Phosphorus | 83 mg |
| Fat | 0.5% | Iron | 25.5 mg |
| Minerals | 2.7% | Vitamin C | 99 mg |
| Fibre | 1.0% | Small amount of | |
| | | Vitamin B Complex | |
| Carbohydrates | 6.1% | | |
| | 100% | | |

*Values per 100 gms edible portions          **Calorific Value - 45**

## Natural Benefits and Curative Properties

Regular use of amaranth in our food items prevents the deficiency of vitamins A, $B_1$, $B_2$, and C, calcium, iron and potassium. It protects against several disorders such as defective vision, respiratory infections, recurrent colds retarded growth and functional sterility.

## Respiratory Disorders

Amaranth is valuable in respiratory system disorders. Drink-

ing fresh juice along with honey is remedy for chronic bronchi
tis, asthma, emphysema and tuberculosis [1]

## Pregnancy and Lactation

Regular use of amaranth during pregnancy and lactation is
highly beneficial One cup of fresh leaf juice of amaranth mixed
with honey and a pinch of cardamom powder should be taken
during the entire period of pregnancy It will help the normal
growth of the baby, prevent the loss of calcium and iron from the
body, relax the uterine ligaments and facilitate easy delivery
without much pain Its use after child birth will shorten the
laying-in period, check the postnatal complications, and
increase the flow of breast milk.[2]

## Retarded Growth

Amaranth is very useful in preventing retarded growth in
children. A teaspoonful of the fresh juice mixed with few drops
of honey should be given once every day to infants after a fort
night of the birth It will help the baby to grow healthy and
strong It will prevent constipation and ease the teething process
as the baby grows

Growing children can safely be given this juice as a natural
protein tonic It contains all the essential amino-acids such as
arginine, histidine, isoleucine, leucine, lysine, cystine, methio-
nine, phenylalanine, threonine, tryptophan and valine

## Premature Ageing

The regular use of amaranth is useful in preventing prema
ture old age It prevents the disturbance of calcium and iron
metabolism which usually occurs in old age. According to Dr.
Van-Sylke, calcium molecules begin to get deposited in the bone
tissues as one becomes old This haphazard calcium distribution
is influenced by the improper molecular movements of iron in
the tissues. If this molecular disturbance of calcium and iron is
prevented by regular supply of food calcium and iron as found
in amaranth and the health is maintained by its regular use from
the early age, the process of ageing can be prevented

## Bleeding Tendencies

The use of amaranth is valuable in all bleeding tendencies. A

1. Dr. Aman, *Medicinal Secrets of Your Foods,* p 316, Indo-
American Hospital, Mysore, 1985
2. Ibid, p.317

cupful of fresh leaf juice mixed with a teaspoonful of lime juice should be taken every night in conditions like bleeding from the gums, nose, lungs, piles and excessive menstruation. It acts as a natural tonic.

**Leucorrhoea**

Amaranth is beneficial in the treatment of leucorrhoea. The rind of the root of amaranth rubbed in 250 ml. of water and strained. It should be given to the patient daily in the morning as well as in the evening. It is a very effective remedy for this disease and quite often the very first dose gives relief. The root of amaranth is very much susceptible to moths. Hence care should be taken to see that it is not moth-eaten. In case good root is not available, its leaves and branches may be used.[3]

# Asparagus

Botanical Name : *Asparagus officinalis*
Indian Name : *Shatwār, Soot mooli and Halyan*

**Description**

The asparagus is cultivated mostly for its tender shoots, commonly known as spears. This vegetable is of great importance in the diet because of its valuable salts, vitamins and for its large amount of cellulose contents. The asparagus is a perennial plant, with underground fleshy root-stock. The young shoots are eaten when 6 to 15 cm. high.

**Origin and Distribution**

Asparagus is native of the eastern Mediterranean lands and Asia Minor. The Romans cultivated the plant in 200 BC. It has, over the centuries, been taken into gardens from the wild and progressively improved by selection. In China, there are several wild species; the tuberous roots of some of which are used as food as well as in medicine. Asparagus is now an important crop, espe-

3. Kvj. Ganpati Singh Verma, *Miracles of Indian Herbs,* p. 109, The Rasayan Pharmacy, New Delhi, Third Edition. 1970.

cially in Taiwan where the shoots are canned for export. It is widely grown in East Africa and Malaysia.

**Asparagus***

| Food Value | | Minerals and Vitamins | |
|---|---|---|---|
| Moisture | 93.0% | Calcium | 22 mg |
| Protein | 2.2% | Phosphorus | 62 mg |
| Fat | 0.2% | Magnesium | 20 mg |
| Fibre | 0.7% | Iron | 1.0 mg |
| Carbohydrates | 3.9% | Vitamin A | 900 IU |
| | 100% | Vitamin C | 33 mg |
| | | Small amount of | |
| | | Vitamin B Complex | |

*Values per 100 gms edible portions          **Calorific Value - 59**

## Natural Benefits and Curative Properties

The asparagus has multipurpose therapeutic properties. It is an alkaline foodstuff. It is an excellent body cleanser and its use will prevent or combat blood acidity. It has a nitrogenous content called 'asparagin' which has diuretic properties. It is said that the liberal use of the young shoots acts as a rejuvenator. However, the use of asparagus should be avoided in goitre, liver and kidney diseases and in case of excess mucus, especially cetarrhal mucus.[1]

### Rheumatism

The asparagus is a valuable food medicine in rheumatism on account of its potash content. But it should be steamed and not boiled as in boiling about four-fifths of the valuable salts are lost. An infusion prepared from this vegetable is also considered highly beneficial in the treatment of rheumatism and chronic gout. It should be given in doses of 30 to 60 ml. It should, however, be avoided in advanced stages of kidney diseases.[2]

### Heart Disease

The asparagus is an excellent food for strengthening the heart. A food medicine for weak or enlarged hearts is prepared by mixing the freshly expressed juice of this vegetable with honey

---

1. Lelord Kordel, *Health the Easy Way*, p. 131, Award Book, New York, 1976.
2. Dr. S.J. Singh, *Food Remedies* p. 25, Nature Cure Council of Medical Research, Lucknow, 1982.

and taking a teaspoonful three times daily. Patients with heart disease will also benefit by eating the cooked vegetable provided the cooking is done conservatively, preferably in steamed form.

**Sexual Debility**

The dried roots of asparagus are used in Unani medicine as an aphrodisiac which arouses sexual desire. It is available in the market as *Safed musli*. Roots boiled in milk are used as demulcent or soothing medicine. Its regular use thickens the semen and is valuable in impotency.

# *Beet Root*

Botanical Name : *Beta vulgaris*
Indian Name : *Chukandar*

**Description**

The red beet, commonly known as garden beet, is a juicy root vegetable. It is distinguished by its individual flavour. It is more colourful than other root vegetables. Beets have several varieties, which are grouped according to their shapes. They are flat, short-top shaped, deep oblate to round, globular to oval, half long and long  The two varieties, most commonly grown in India are Crimson Globe and Detriot Dark Red, both belonging to the globular to oval group

**Origin and Distribution**

Beet is believed to be a native of the Mediterranean region of Europe or around West Asia. It has been used as a vegetable for the last 2,000 years, even by early Greeks and Romans. It is now widely distributed in the tropics and is cultivated in the Caribbean, Malaysia, Indonesia, Philippines, Central, East and West Africa. In India it is cultivated for its nutritious roots.

**Food Value**

This vegetable is a good tonic food for health. It contains carbohydrates, mainly in the form of sugar, and it has a little protein and fat. Beet is taken in a variety of ways. They are widely used in salads and in the preparation of pickles and chutney. They are also baked like potatoes or boiled, steamed or cooked

They should be thoroughly washed before boiling and the skin should be removed before use. The leaves, like all green vegetables, should be cooked with a small amount of water and for only a short time. The fresher the beets, the better the flavour and the quicker they cook.

**Beet Root***

| Food Value | | Minerals and Vitamins | |
|---|---|---|---|
| Moisture | 87.7% | Calcium | 18 mg |
| Protein | 1.7% | Phosphorus | 55 mg |
| Fat | 0.1% | Iron | 1.0 mg |
| Minerals | 0.8% | Vitamin C | 10 mg |
| Fibre | 0.9% | Good amount of Vitamin | |
| Carbohydrates | 8.8% | A & B and small amount | |
| | 100% | of Vitamin B complex | |

*Values per 100 gms edible portions      **Calorific Value** 43

The beet juice is considered as one of the best vegetable juice. It is a rich source of natural sugar. It contains sodium, potassium, phosphorus, calcium, sulphur, chlorine, iodine, iron, copper, vitamin $B_1$, $B_2$, niacin, $B_6$, C and P. This juice is rich in easily digestible carbohydrates, but the calorie content is low. The protein factors or amino acids are good in both quality and quantity.

## Natural Benefits and Curative Properties

Beets are of great therapeutic value. They have properties to clean the kidneys and gall bladder. Being rich in alkaline elements, potassium, calcium, magnesium and iron, they are useful in combating acidosis and aid the natural processes of elimination.

### Anaemia

Red beet juice is associated with human blood and blood forming qualities. Due to its higher content of iron, it regenerates and reactivates the red blood cells, supplies fresh oxygen to the body and helps the normal function of vesicular breathing i.e. normal breath sound. It is thus extremely useful in the treatment of anaemia.

According to Dr. Fritz Keitel of Germany, "The juice of the

red beet strengthens the body's powers of resistance and has proved to be an excellent remedy for anaemia, especially for children and teenagers where other blood forming remedies have failed" [1]

## Digestive Disorders

Beet juice is beneficial in the treatment of jaundice, hepatitis, nausea and vomiting due to biliousness, diarrhoea and dysentary Adding a teaspoonful of lime juice to this juice increases its medicinal value and can be given as a liquid food in these conditions. Fresh beet juice mixed with a tablespoonful of honey taken every morning before breakfast helps the healing of gastric ulcer. [2]

Leaves of beet root, eaten as green-leafy vegetable and its juice, mixed with lime juice, are also valuable in jaundice and gastric ulcer. The juice should be taken once daily.

## Constipation and Piles

The cellulose content of the beet acts as a bulk residue, increases peristalsis—i.e. wavelike movement and eases the passage of stool. Its regular use thus prevents habitual constipation. A decoction of the beet root is highly valuable in chronic constipation and haemorrhoids, i.e. piles. It may be given in doses of half to one tumblerful at bed time.

## Circulatory Disorders

The beet juice is an excellent solvent for inorganic calcium deposits. It is, therefore, valuable in the treatment of hypertension, arteriosclerosis, heart trouble and varicose veins

## Kidney and Gall Bladder Disorders

The beet juice, in combination with the juice of carrot and cucumber, is one of the finest cleansing material for kidneys and gall bladder. It is highly beneficial in all disorders relating to these two organs.

## Skin Disorders

The water in which beet roots and tops have been boiled is an excellent application for boils, skin inflammation and out breaks of pimples and pustules. The white beet is better for this

1. Linda Clark, *Handbook of Natural Remedies for Common Ail ments*, p. 44, Pocket Books, New York, 1976.
2. N.W. Walker, *Raw Vegetable Juices*, p 34, Jove Books, New York, 1983

purpose. For an irritable skin the body should be sponged down occasionally with a mixture of three parts of beet water to one part of white vinegar. This mixture is also useful as a skin wash in cases of measles and eruptive fevers.

**Dandruff**

The decoction of beets mixed with little vinegar can be used externally to cleanse scurf or dandruff from the head. For dandruff, the beet water should also be massaged into the scalp with the ginger tip every night.

# *Bitter Gourd*

Botanical Name : *Monordica charantia*
Other English Names : *Bitter cucumber, Bitter melon and Balsam pear*
Indian Name : *Karelā*

**Description**

The bitter gourd is a common vegetable cultivated extensively all over India. It is 10 to 20 cm. long, tapering at the ends and covered with blunt tubercles The seeds are white in raw fruits and become red when they are ripe. There are two varieties of this vegetable. The large kind is long, oblong and pale green in colour. The other kind is small, little oval and dark green. Both the types are bitter in taste. They turn reddish-orange when ripe.

**Origin and Distribution**

### Bitter Gourd*

| Food Value | | Minerals and Vitamins | |
|---|---|---|---|
| Moisture | 92.4% | Calcium | 20 mg |
| Protein | 1.6% | Phosphorus | 70 mg |
| Fat | 0.2% | Iron | 1.8 mg |
| Minerals | 0.8% | Vitamin C | 88 mg |
| Fibre | 0.8% | Small amount of | |
| Carbohydrates | 4.2% | Vitamin B Complex | |
| | 100% | | |

*Values per 100 gms edible portion          **Calorific Value - 25**

94

The original home of bitter gourd is not known except that it is a native of the tropics. It is widely grown in India, Indonesia, Sri Lanka, Malaysia, the Philippines, China and the Caribbean.

## Natural Benefits and Curative Properties

The bitter gourd has excellent medicinal virtues. It is antidotal, antipyretic tonic, appetizing, stomachic, antibilious and laxative.[1] The bitter gourd is also used in native medicines of Asia and Africa.

### Diabetes

The bitter gourd is specifically used as a folk medicine for diabetes. Recent researches by a team of British doctors have established that it contains a hypoglycaemic or insulin-like principle, designated as 'plant-insulin', which has been found highly beneficial in lowering the blood and urine sugar levels. It should, therefore, be included liberally in the diet of the diabetic. For better results, the diabetic should take the juice of about four or five fruits every morning on an empty stomach. The seeds of bitter gourd can be added to food in the powdered form. Diabetics can also use bitter gourd in the form of decoction by boiling the pieces in water or in the form of dry powder.

A mojority of diabetics usually suffer from malnutrition as they are usually under-nourished. Bitter gourd being rich in all the essential vitamins and minerals, especially vitamin A, $B_1$, $B_2$, C and Iron, its regular use prevents many complications such as hypertension, eye complications, neuritis and defective metabolism of carbohydrates. It increases body's resistance against infection.

### Piles

Juice of the fresh leaves of bitter gourd is valuable in piles. Three teaspoonfuls of leaf juice mixed with a glassful of buttermilk should be taken every morning for about a month in this condition. A paste of the roots of bitter gourd plant can also be applied over piles with beneficial results.

### Blood Disorders

Bitter gourd is highly beneficial in the treatment of blood disorders like blood boils, scabies, itching, psoriasis, ring-worm

---

1. J.F. Dastur, *Medicinal Plants of India and Pakistan,* p. 112, D.B. Taraporevala Sons & Co. (P) Ltd., Bombay, 1985.

and other fungal diseases. A cupful of fresh juice of bitter gourd mixed with a teaspoonful of lime juice should be taken, sip by sip, on empty stomach daily for four to six months in these conditions. Its regular use in endemic regions of leprosy acts as a preventive medicine.[2]

### Respiratory Disorders

Bitter gourd plant roots are used in folk medicine for respiratory disorders from ancient times. A teaspoonful of the root paste mixed with equal amount of honey or *tulsi* leaf juice, given once every night for a month acts as an excellent medicine for asthma, bronchitis, pharyngitis, colds and rhinitis

### Alcoholism

Leaf juice is beneficial in the treatment of alcoholism. It is an antidote for alcohol intoxication. It is also useful in liver dam age due to alcoholism

### Cholera

Fresh juice of leaves of bitter gourd is also an effective medi cine in early stages of cholera and other types of diarrhoea during summer  Two teaspoonfuls of this juice mixed with equal quantity of white onion juice and a teaspoonful of lime juice should be given in these conditions.

### Uses

The bitter gourd is cooked and eaten as a vegetable in India and the Far East. The bitterness is reduced by steeping the peeled fruit in salt water before cooking. It is also used in pickles and as an ingredient of curries. The seeds of the ripe fruit are used as a condiment in India. The tender shoots and leaves are used as spinach.

# *Bottle Gourd*

Botanical Name : *Lagenaria vulgaris*
Other English Names : *White gourd, Trumpet gourd*
Indian Name : *Lauki, Doodhi, Ghia and Kaddu*

### Description

The bottle gourd is a common vegetable in India. It is yellow-

2. S.A Majeed, *Tibbe-Rahamani*, Urdu, p. 118, 1928,

ish green, having the shape of a bottle. It has white pulp, with white seeds embedded in spongy flesh.

## Origin and Distribution

The bottle gourds have been cultivated since time immemorial and they are, probably one of the earliest vegetables cultivated by man. It appears to have originated in Africa where it occurs spontaneously as it also does in India. It is now widely cultivated throughout the tropics, especially India, Sri Lanka, Indonesia, Malaysia, the Philippines, China, tropical Africa and South America. The bottle gourd is a warm season crop and grows best in a warm humid climate.

**Bottle Gourd***

| Food Value | | Minerals and Vitamins | |
|---|---|---|---|
| Moisture | 96.1% | Calcium | 20 mg |
| Protein | 0.2% | Phosphorus | 10 mg |
| Fat | 0.1% | Iron | 0.7 mg |
| Minerals | 0.5% | Small amount of | |
| Fibre | 0.6% | Vitamin B Complex | |
| Carbohydrates | 2.5% | | |
| | 100% | | |

*Values per 100 gms edible portion     **Calorific Value - 12**

## Natural Benefits and Curative Properties

The cooked vegetable is cooling, diuretic, sedative and antibilious. It gives a feeling of relaxation after eating it. However, bottle gourd should not be eaten in a raw state as it may prove harmful for stomach and intestines.

### Urinary Disorders

Bottle gourd is very valuable in urinary disorders. A glassful of fresh juice prepared by grating the whole fruit should be mixed with teaspoonful of lime juice. It should be given once daily in the treatment of burning sensation in urinary passage due to high acidity of urine. It serves as an alkaline mixture. It should be given with sulpha drugs in the treatment of urinary infection. It acts as an alkaline diuretic in this condition.

### Excessive Thirst

The juice of bottle gourd is a valuable medicine for excessive thirst due to severe diarrhoea, diabetes and excessive use of fatty or fried foods. A glassful of plain juice with a pinch of salt should be taken everyday in this condition. Its use during summer prevents excessive loss of sodium, quenches thirst and helps in preventing fatigue.

**Insomnia**

This mixture of bottle gourd juice and sesame oil acts as an effective medicine for insomnia. It should be massaged over scalp every night. The cooked leaves of bottle gourd are also beneficial in the treatment of insomnia.

# Cabbage

Botanical Names : *Brassica oleracea var, capitata*
Indian Names : *Bandgobhi, Karam kalla and Pattagobhi*

**Description**

The cabbage is one of the most highly rated leafy-vegetables and a marvellous food item. It is grown for its enlarged edible, terminal buds and is eaten all over the world. It is excellent as a muscle builder and cleanser. There are several varieties of cabbage. They differ in size, shape and colour of leaves, and in size, shape, colour and texture of head.

**Origin and Distribution**

The cabbage was cultivated long before the dawn of human history. The ancient Greeks regarded it as an important vegetable. It was also very popular in Rome and it was introduced by the Romans into those lands which they conquered. The original home of cabbage is Southern Europe and the Mediterranean regions. The major areas of cultivation are Northern India, Indonesia, Malaysia, the Philippines, Central, East and West Africa, Central and South America and the Caribbean.

**Food Value**

This vegetable is chiefly valuable for its high mineral and vitamin content and alkaline salts. This vegetable can be used raw in the form of salad. It can also be steamed, boiled or cooked. It should be eaten raw for best results as in cooking its valuable nutrients are largely lost. The raw cabbage is also more easily digested than the cooked one. The longer the cabbage is cooked the less digestible it becomes. It can be rectified by adding some asafoetida i.e. *hing*. The cabbage with green leaves is especially valuable because of its high vitamin A content.

**Cabbage***

| Food Value | | Minerals and Vitamins | |
|---|---|---|---|
| Moisture | 91.9% | Calcium | 39 mg |
| Protein | 1.8% | Phosphorus | 44 mg |
| Fat | 0.1% | Iron | 0.8 mg |
| Minerals | 0.6% | Vitamin C | 124 mg |
| Fibre | 1.0% | Small amount of | |
| Carbohydrates | 4.6% | Vitamin B complex | |
| | 100% | | |

*Values per 100 gms edible portions **Calorific Value - 27**

## Nutural Benefits and Curative Properties

The cabbage has wonderful cleansing and reducing properties. Its most valuable properties are the high sulphur and chlorine content and the relatively large per cent of iodine. The combination of the sulphur and chlorine causes a cleansing of the mucus membranes of the stomach and intestinal tract, but this only applies when cabbage or its juice is taken in its raw state without the addition of salt.

However, cabbage and cabbage juice should never be taken as a main part of the diet. Very excessive intakes have been known to cause the thyroid disease called goitre. It is only in normal amounts that cabbage is valuable nutritionally and that its juice, which is bitter and not delicious, constitutes an important part of the natural treatment of infection, ulcers and other disorders of the digestive system.[1]

### Constipation

The cabbage provides the roughage i.e., indigestible material which is essential to stimulate intestines for the proper action of the bowels. A meal of raw cabbage is an excellent remedy for constipation. It acts immediately without any adverse after-effects. This meal can be prepared by adding a little salt, black

---

1. Susane E. Charmine, *The Complete Raw Juice Therapy*, p. 59, Thorsons Publishing Group, Great Britain, 1987.

pepper and lemon juice to finely chopped raw cabbage.

## Stomach Ulcers

Duodenal ulcers have responded almost miraculously to the drinking of cabbage juice. Its origin as a traditional remedy goes back to the work of Garnet Cheney, M.D., of Stanford University School of Medicine some thirty years back. He is reported to have cured many ulcer patients with raw cabbage juice. The juice contains the antiulcer factor, vitamin U. This vitamin is destroyed by cooking. The treatment consists of taking 90 to 180 gm. of cabbage juice for three times daily followed by a natural diet.

To render the juice more palatable Dr. Cheney often added celery juice, made from both stalk and green, pineapple juice, tomato juice or citrus juice. Chilling the mixed juice also helps to improve the flavour. The juice, however, should not be taken all at once, but in many intervals throughout the day. If one does not have a juicer or blender, one can nibble on raw cabbage four or five times a day.[2]

## Obesity

Recent research has discovered in cabbage a valuable content called tartronic acid which inhibits the conversion of sugar and other carbohydrates into fat. Hence, it is of great value in weight reduction. Taking cabbage salad would be the simplest way to stay slim, a painless way of dieting.

A hundred grams of cabbage yields only 27 kilocalories of energy while the same quantity of wheat bread will yield about 240 calories. Cabbage is found to posses the maximum biological value with minimum calorific value. Moreover, it gives a lasting feeling of fullness in the stomach and is easily digestible.

## Skin Disorders

The cabbage leaves have been successfully used in the form of compresses in healing ulcers, infected sores, blisters and skin eruptions, including psoriasis. They are also valuable in burns and carbuncles. The thickest and greenest outer leaves are most effective for use as compresses. They should be thoroughly washed in warm water and dried with a towel. The whole leaves should be used for large compresses.

---

2. Mark Bricklin, *Rodale's Encyclopedia of Natural Home Remedies*, p. 466, D.B. Taraporevala Son and Co (P) Ltd, Bombay, 1982.

The leaves should be made flat, soft and smooth by rolling them with a rolling pin after removing the thick veins. They should be warmed and then applied smoothly to the affected part in an overlapping manner. The leaves may be cut into thin strips for treating a small area. The cabbage leaves should be placed on a linen cloth and a pad of soft woollen cloth should be put over it. The whole compress should then be secured with an elastic bandage. The compress can be kept for the whole day and night. If, however, the leaves wither or change colour, they should be replaced by fresh ones. When changing the compress, affected area should be thoroughly washed and dried.[3]

## Premature Ageing

Research has shown that cabbage contains several elements and factors which enhance the immunity of the human body and arrests its premature ageing. The vegetable is of great value for persons of advancing age. Some of the elements help prevent the formation of patches on the walls of blood vessels and stones in the gall bladder. It has been found that a combination of vitamin P and C in cabbage lends strength to the blood vessels.

# *Carrot*

Botanical Name : *Daucus carota*
Indian Name : *Gājar*

## Description

The carrot is a popular vegetable the world over. It is a powerful cleansing food. Green carrot leaves are highly nutritive, rich in protein, minerals and vitamins.

There are many varieties of carrot. Broadly, they can be classified into two groups, namely, Asiatic types and European types. The former are marked by their larger size, darker colour and sweet taste. However, the latter are preferred due to the smooth surface, thin core, better shape and being less fibrous in nature.

3. Dr. S. J. Singh, *Food Remedies*, pp. 52-53, *Nature Cure Council of Medical Research, Lucknow, 1982.*

## Origin and Distribution

The carrot appears to have originated in Central Asia, in the hills of Punjab and Kashmir in India, with a secondary centre of distribution in Asia, Europe and North Africa around the Mediterranean. It is cultivated in India, Malaysia, Indonesia, Philippines, Central, East and West Africa, South America and the Caribbean.

## Food Value

Nutritionally, the carrot is an extremely rich source of vitamin A. The name carotene, which is a form of pro-vitamin, has been derived from carrot. The carotene is converted into vitamin A by the liver and it is also stored in our body.

Carrots are rich in sodium, sulphur, chlorine and contain traces of iodine. The mineral contents in carrots lie very close to the skin. Hence they should not be peeled or scrapped off.

### Carrot*

| Food Value | | Minerals and Vitamins | |
|---|---|---|---|
| Carrot | 86.0% | Calcium | 80 mg |
| Protein | 0.9% | Phosphorus | 530 mg |
| Fat | 0.2% | Iron | 2.2 mg |
| Minerals | 1.1% | Vitamin C | 3 mg |
| Fibre | 1.2% | Small amount of | |
| Carbohydrates | 10.6% | Vitamin B Complex | |
| | 100% | | |

*Values per 100 gms edible portion      **Calorific Value** -48

## Natural Benefits and Curative Properties

Carrot is rich in alkaline elements which purify and revitalise the blood. It nourishes the entire system and helps in the maintenance of acid-alkaline balance in the body.

The juice of carrot is known as a "Miracle Juice". It makes a fine health-giving drink for children and adults alike. It strengthens the eyes and keeps the mucus membranes of all cavities of the body in healthy condition. It is beneficial in the treatment of dry and rough skin.

However, the use of carrot seeds should be avoided during early period of pregnancy, because it increases the toxicity of uterine walls and may cause abortion.

102

## Tooth Decay

Chewing a carrot immediately after food kills all the harmful germs in the mouth. It cleans the teeth, removes the food particles lodged in the crevices and prevents bleeding of the gums and tooth decay.

## Digestive Disorders

Chewing of carrots increases saliva and quickens digestion by supplying the necessary enzymes, minerals and vitamins. Regular use of carrot prevents the formation of gastric ulcer and other digestive disorders. Carrot juice is an effective food remedy in ailments like intestinal colic, colitis, appendicitis, peptic ulcer and dyspepsia.

## Constipation

Carrot juice, combined with spinach juice and a little lemon juice, is very effective in the treatment of constipation. Spinach juice cleanses the bowels. This effect cannot be expected soon after taking the juice. But within two months, the bowel starts emptying regularly. About 50 ml. of spinach juice should be added to 250 ml. of carrot juice to make this combination.

## Diarrhoea

The carrot soup has been found an effective natural remedy for diarrhoea. It supplies fluid to combat dehydration, replenishes sodium, potassium, phosphorus, calcium, sulphur and magnesium. It is a good source of pectin and coats the intestines to allay imflammation. It checks the growth of harmful bacteria and prevents vomiting. It is especially useful for children. ½ Kg. of carrot may be cooked in 150 ml. of water until it is soft. The pulp should be strained. Three-quarter tablespoon of salt may be added and a small amount of the soup should be given to the patient every half an hour. Improvement is usually noticeable in 24 hours.[1]

## Thread Worms

The carrots are valuable in the elimination of thread worms from children as it is offensive to all parasites. A small cupful of grated carrot taken every morning, with no other food added to the meal, can clear these worms quickly.

Raw carrots are good for fertility. Sterility is sometimes

1. Linda Clark, *Handbook of Natural Remedies for Common Ailments*, p. 131, Pocket Books, New York, 1977.

overcome by its use. The cause of sterility has been traced to the continuous use of food in which enzmes are destroyed by cooking or pasteurizing.

## Uses

Carrots can be used in a variety of way. They may be eaten raw in salads, or they may be boiled or cooked. They can also be used in the form of soup and juice. They are most helpful when they are taken raw. In cooking, a large amount of the important minerals are lost. They form very important ingredient of a raw salad.

# *Cucumber*

Botanical Name : *Cucumis sativas*
Indian Name : *Khirā*

## Description

The cucumber is a very popular and widely cultivated vegetable in India. It gives cooling and refreshing effect. It contains almost all the essential elements needed for the preservation of health.

There are several varieties of cucumber which differ in shape, size and colour. Its colour varies from whitish green to dark green. It turns into orange, yellow or brownish yellow when it matures. Its sizes also vary from 8 to 30 cm. and above. Fresh, firm, smooth, regular in shape and dark green in colour is the best variety for use.

## Origin and Distribution

Cucumber is believed to have originated in northern India. It was known to ancient Egyptians, Greeks and Romans and was available in China in the sixth century AD. It has now spread throughout the world. Its areas of cultivation include northern and southern India, South East Asia, China, Africa, central and South America, the Caribbean and most tropical areas.

## Food Value

Nutritionaliy, the cucumber has a relatively high mineral

content. Its skin is most valuable as the cell salts and vitamins are in and near it. Hence it should not be peeled.

It is also a valuable source of potassium, sodium, magnesium, sulphur, silicon, chlorine and fluorine. The cucumber taken with vegetables, cereals, fruits, nuts and salads enhances the nutritional value of food items. It is generally used as a salad in combination with carrot, beet, tomato, radish, lettuce and other vegetables. The addition of some curd to the salad will make it a tasty food of great nutritional value.

**Cucumber***

| Food Value | | Minerals and Vitamins | |
|---|---|---|---|
| Moisture | 96.3% | Calcium | 10 mg |
| Protein | 0.4% | Phosphorus | 25 mg |
| Fat | 0.1% | Iron | 1.5 mg |
| Minerals | 0.3% | Vitamin C | 7 mg |
| Fibre | 0.4% | Small amount of | |
| Carbohydrates | 2.5% | Vitamin B Complex | |
| | 100% | | |

*Values per 100 gms edible portion          **Calorific Value - 13**

## Natural Benefits and Curative Properties

The alkaline-forming minerals in the cucumber represent 64.05 per cent and the acid-forming minerals 35.95 per cent. This mineral arrangement invests the cucumber with definite remedial and curative properties. It makes it useful in maintaining the alkalinity of the blood. It also operates as one of the best natural diuretics, secreting and promoting the flow of urine. It should always be taken raw as in cooking potassium and phosphorus are lost.

### Constipation

The cucumber is a dependable laxative food. It supplies bulk to aid bowel action. Those who suffer from constipation can greatly benefit by taking two cucumbers a day.

### Stomach Disorders

The juice of the cucumber is a valuable food medicine in the treatment of hyperacidity, gastric and duodenal ulcers. It should be taken in doses of four to six ounces every two hours in such conditions. Sufficient juice can be extracted from a cucumber as it contains 96 per cent water. It gives immediate relief when there is a burning sensation in the stomach.

## Rheumatic Ailments

Cucumber juice in combination with the juice of carrots, beets and celery, has a very beneficial effect in the conditions associated with accumulation of uric acid such as arthritis, gout and rheumatism.

## Urinary Disorders

Cucumber seeds are rich in potassium. Emulsion of the shelled seeds has been found highly beneficial in the treatment of burning sensation in urinary calculi or stone in persons who are predisposed to such disorders. Emulsion of the shelled seeds, mixed with curd, is useful in dissolving the gravel in urinary tract and in reducing hyperacidity of the urine.[1]

## Cholera

A glassful of fresh leaf juice mixed with tender coconut water, given one or two ounces every hour, is a medicine for excessive thirst during cholera. It acts excellently by restoring the electrolyte liquid balance in dehydration.

## Skin Eruptions

Cucumber juice has proved effective in skin eruption. For better results, juices of carrot, lettuce should be added to this juice. Further, addition of little alfalfa juice in some cases can help to speed up their efficacy.

## Beauty Aid

Grated cucumber applied over face, eyes and neck for 15 to 20 minutes has been found effective as a beauty aid and a best tonic for the skin of the face. Its regular use prevents pimples, blackheads, wrinkles and dryness of the face. Cucumber juice promotes hair growth due to its high silicon and sulphur content, particularly when mixed with carrot, lettuce and spinach juice.

---

1. Dr. Aman, *Medicinal Secrets of Your Food*, p. 426, Indo American Hospital, Mysore, 1985

# Drumstick

Botanical Name : *Moringa oleifera*
Indian Name : *Sanjanā*

## Description

The drumstick is a fairly common vegetable grown all over India and Pakistan. It is valued mainly for the tender pod. It is antibacterial and a wonderful cleanser.

The drumstick tree is perennial, erect, slender, medium sized with many arching branches. It is mostly grown as a backyard tree in most of the South Indian homes. It has drumstick like fruits, small white flowers and small and round leaves which are cooked and eaten as vegetable.

## Food Value

Nutritionally, drumstick pods and leaves are of great value as sources of acrotene, calcium, phosphorus and vitamin C. The leaves, flowers and fruits of drumstick which are used as vegetable have great nutritional value. The tender fruit is used in

### Drumstick (Pods)*

| Food Value | | Minerals and Vitamins | |
|---|---|---|---|
| Moisture | 86.9% | Calcium | 30 mg |
| Protein | 2.5% | Phosphorus | 110 mg |
| Fat | 0.1% | Iron | 5.3 mg |
| Minerals | 2.0% | Vitamin C | 120 mg |
| Fibre | 4.8% | Small amount of | |
| Carbohydrates | 3.7% | Vitamin B Complex | |
| | 100% | | |

Calorific Value - 26

### Drumstick (Leaves)*

| Food Value | | Minerals and Vitamins | |
|---|---|---|---|
| Moisture | 75.9% | Calcium | 440 mg |
| Protein | 6.7% | Phosphorus | 70 mg |
| Fat | 1.7% | Iron | 7 mg |
| Minerals | 2.3% | Vitamin C | 220 mg |
| Fibre | 0.9% | Small amount of | |
| Carbohydrates | 12.5% | Vitamin B complex | |
| | 100% | | |

*Values per 100 gms edible portion          Calorific Value - 92

*samber* and most dishes in South Indian homes. The leaves and flowers are used to prepare curry and cake.

## Natural Benefits and Curative Properties

Almost all parts of the drumstick tree have therapeutic value. The leaves are especially beneficial in the treatment of many ailments due to their various medicinal properties and their rich iron content. They are used as food also.

### Tonic for Children

The leaves serve as a tonic for infants and growing children. For better results, juice should be extracted from leaves, filtered and mixed with milk. This mixture becomes an excellent tonic for healthy and strong bones and for purifying bloodstream.

### Pregnancy and Lactation

Taking this tonic regularly by expectant mothers will provide them with necessary calcium, iron and vitamins. It will also help them overcome sluggishness of the uterus, facilitate easy delivery and reduce post delivery complications. A vegetable prepared from leaves increases breast milk after child birth. This vegetable is prepared by boiling the leaves with salt and water. The water is then drained off and they are smeared with ghee and eaten.

### Respiratory Disorder

A soup prepared from drumstick leaves is highly beneficial in the treatment of respiratory diseases like asthma, bronchitis and tuberculosis. This soup is prepared by adding a handful of leaves to 180 ml. of water and is allowed to boil for five minutes. It should then be allowed to cool. A little salt, pepper and lime juice may be added to this soup.[1]

### Infections

Drumstick soup made with leaves and flowers as well as boiled drumsticks are highly valuable in preventing infections of all kinds such as that of the throat, chest and skin. This is because drumstick has antibacterial properties very much like penicillin and other antibiotics.

### Sexual Disorders

A soup made with drumstick flowers boiled in milk is very

1. Dr. Aman, *Medicinal Secrets of Your Food*, p. 341, Indo-American Hospital, Mysore, 1985.

useful as a sexual tonic in the treatment of sexual debility. It is also useful in functional sterility in both males and females.

The powder of the dry bark is valuable in impotency, premature ejaculation and thinness of semen. About 120 gm. of the powder of the dry bark should be boiled in 600 ml. of water for about half an hour and 30 ml. of this. mixed with a table spoonful of honey, should be taken three times daily for a month to cure these conditions.[2]

### Digestive Disorders

Drumstick is also valuable in digestive disorders. A teaspoonful of fresh leaf juice, mixed with honey and a glassful of tender coconut water, is given two or three times as a herbal-medicine during the treatment of cholera, dysentery, diarrhoea, colitis and jaundice.

### Urinary Disorders

A tablespoonful of coagulated fresh leaf juice, mixed with a glass of fresh juice of cucumber or carrot, is an effective medicine for scanty urination and constant burning in urethra due to high acidity of urine. A teaspoonful of the juice with 10 gm. of rocksalt once daily, is used to cure excessive urination of non-diabetics.[3]

### Beauty-Aid

Fresh leaf juice applied with lime juice is useful in the treatment of pimples, black heads and keeps one's face fresh.

# *Fenugreek*

Botanical Name : *Trigonella foenum-graecum*
Indian Name : *Methi*

### Description

Fenugreek is a well-known leafy vegetable. It has excellent medicinal virtues. It is Nature's great boon to mankind and its regular use will help keep the body healthy.

2. Ibid., pp. 343-344.
3. Ibid., p. 342.

Fenugreek is an erect, strongly scented, robust, annual herb, about 30 to 60 cm. high. It has compound leaves of light green colour 2 to 2.5 cm. long, auxiliary yellow flowers, and thin pointed pods, 5 to 7 cm. long. The seeds are brownish yellow and emit peculiar odour.

There are two popular varieties of fenugreek known as *Masuri Methi* or *Champa Methi* and *Marwari Methi*. Both the varieties are scented and are recommended for cultivation.

## Origin and Distribution

Fenugreek is considered to be a native of eastern Europe and Ethopia. It is also found growing wild in north-western India. It has been used since ancient times both as a food and medicine by the people living on the shores of Mediterranean and in Asia. The fenugreek is a cool season crop and it grows all over India.

## Food Value

In India, the plants and leaves of fenugreek known as *methi-ka-saag* are commonly used as culinary vegetables. Steaming is considered the best method of cooking leaves as in this process the vitamins are retained and the vegetable is palatable. The dried leaves can be compared to pulses for their protein content. They supplement the lysine-deficient cereal diets. Lysine is amino acid which is fundamental constituents of all proteins. The seeds of fenugreek contain a foetid and bitter fatty oil resin, mucilage and albumin. Their mineral and vitamin contents are very high. In Indian homes, seeds are generally used as a condiment and for flavouring.

### Fenugreek*

| Food Value | | Minerals and Vitamins | |
|---|---|---|---|
| Moisture | 86.1% | Calcium | 395 mg |
| Protein | 4.4% | Phosphorus | 51 mg |
| Fat | 0.9% | Iron | 16.5 mg |
| Minerals | 1.5% | Vitamin C | 52 mg |
| Fibre | 1.1% | Small amount of | |
| Carbohydrates | 6.0% | Vitamin B Complex | |
| | 100% | | |

*Value per 100 gms edible portion  **Calorific Value - 49**

## Natural Benefits and Curative Properties

The leaves of fenugreek are aromatic, cooling and mild aperient. Paste of the fresh leaves applied over the scalp regularly, before taking bath, lengthens hair, preserves the natural colour and keeps the hair silky soft. Paste of the fresh leaves, applied on the face every night before going to bed and washed with warm water, prevents pimples, blackheads, dryness of the face and early appearance of wrinkles. It improves complexion and makes one look years younger. The seeds of fenugreek are demulcent, diuretic, carminative which relieves gastric discomforts, lactagogue, which increases the flow of milk, astringent and aphrodisiac tonic.[1] They are the best cleansers to body, highly mucus-solvents and soothing agents. The seeds are used in the preparation of hair tonics and cosmetics in Java.

### Digestive Disorders

Fenugreek leaves are highly beneficial in the treatment of indigestion, flatulence and sluggish liver. They help in the healing of mouth ulcers. An infusion of the leaves is used as a gargle for recurrent ulcers. Boiled and fried in butter, they are valuable in biliousness. The seeds are also useful in the treatment of colic, flatulence, dysentery, diarrhoea, and dyspepsia.

### Anaemia

The leaves help in blood formation. The cooked leaves are extremely useful for adolescent girls to prevent anaemia and run down condition which is generally associated with the onset of puberty and sudden spurt of growth. The seeds of fenugreek are also valuable in anaemia, being rich in iron.

### Pregnancy and Lactation

The seeds are fried in ghee and finely powdered. This powder is mixed with wheat flour and sugar to prepare a *halwa*. This preparation, taken in small quantity daily, helps in quick normalisation after delivery. The seeds, made into a gruel, are given as diet to nursing mothers for increasing the flow of milk.

### Deadened Sense of Taste and Smell

The seeds help restore a deadened sense of taste or smell. The loss of sense of taste occurs due to improper functioning of the salivary glands. They often become plugged with mucus and accumulated juices, causing swelling. Similarly, the sense of smell is obstructed due to long accumulations of mucus or other

---

1. J.F. Dastur, *Medicinal Plants of India and Pakistan,* p. 169, D.B. Taraporevala Sons & Co. (P) Ltd., Bombay, 1985.

impurities in the nose where the olfactory nerves are based. Regular use of fenugreek has proved beneficial in both these cases.

**Dandruff**

Fenugreek seeds are useful in the removal of dandruff. Two tablespoonfuls of the seeds should be soaked overnight in water. In the morning the softened seeds should be ground into a fine paste. This paste should be applied all over the scalp and left on the head for half an hour. The hair should then be washed thoroughly with soapnut solution or shikakai. Paste of the fresh leaves of fenugreek applied over the scalp regularly before taking bath also cures dandruff.

**Fevers**

A tea made from fenugreek seeds is equal in value to quinine for reducing fevers. It is particularly valuable as a cleansing and soothing drink. The fenugreek seeds, when moistened with water are themselves slightly mucilageous. A tea made from them has the power to dissolve more sticky substance as body mucus.

**Stomach Disorders**

The fenugreek tea soothes inflamed stomach and intestines and cleanses the stomach, bowels, kidneys and respiratory tract of excess mucus. It is beneficial in the healing of peptic ulcers as the mild coating of gum like lubricant material deposited by fenugreek, as it passes through the stomach and intestines, provides a protective shell for the ulcers.[2]

**Respiratory Infections**

During the early acute stages of any of the respiratory tract infections, such as bronchitis, influenza, sinusities, catarrah and suspected pneumonia, fenugreek tea will help the body to produce perspiration, dispel toxicity and shorten the period of fever. It should be taken upto four cups daily. The quantity is reduced as condition improves. To improve flavour, a few drops of lemon juice can be used. During such treatment, no form of food or nourishment should be taken as is followed during fasting and fenugreek will allow the body to correct these respiratory problems in a few days.

---

2. Lelord Kordel, *Health The Easy Way,* p. 48, Award Books, New York, 1976.

## Sore Throat

The gargle made from fenugreek seeds is the best for ordi
sore throat. When preparing a gargle, the solution shoul
much stronger than a tea. Two tablespoonfuls of fenugreek seeds
should be put into a quart of cold water and allowed to simmer
for half an hour over a low flame. It should be allowed to cool to
a bearable temperature. It should then be strained and entire
quantity used as a gargle.

## Bad breath and Body Odour

The tea made from fenugreek is also beneficial in the case of
bad breath and body odour. The unpleasant odours emanate
from body openings due to accumulations of hardened mucus
and other toxic substances in the nasal and oral passages, the
gastrointestinal tract, the urinary tract, the bloodstream and
vagina. The fenugreek tea, taken regularly will help remove
these accumulation from such spots where mouth wash and
soap can never penetrate.

## Diabetes

Fenugreek seeds have been found highly effective in the
treatment of diabetes. According to a recent report brought out
by the Indian Council of Medical Research, as quoted by Press
Trust of India on January 6, 1988, fenugreek seeds, when given
in varying doses of 25 grams to 100 grams daily, diminish reac-
tive hyperglycaemia in diabetic patients. Levels of glucose,
serum cholesterol and tryglycerides were also significantly
reduced in the diabetes patients when the seeds were consumed,
the report said Quoting researchers at the National Institute of
Nutrition, Hyderabad, the report said that the effect of taking
fenugreek seeds could be quite dramatic, when consumed with
1200-1400 calories diet per day, which is usually recommended
for diabetic patients.

## Swellings

Due to their cooling properties, a poultice of the leaves can be
applied with advantage in external and internal swellings and
burns.

# Garlic

Botanical Name : *Allium sativum*
Indian Name : *Lahasoon*

## Description

The garlic, a garden vegetable of the onion family, has been cultivated from time immemorial. It has been variously described as a food, a herb, a medicinal plant, an antiseptic a beauty accessory and a magical antidote to evil by various people at different times throughout the ages.

Garlic is an important condiment crop. It is an erect biennial herb normally grown as an annual—i.e. a plant that only lasts for an year. It has adventitious roots and condensed, flattened stem and narrow, flat leaves. The bulb consists of 6 to 35 bulblets called cloves which are enclosed in a thin whitish, glistering and transparent covering.

## Origin and Distribution

The garlic is believed to have originated in Central Asia and was known to the Chinese as early as 3,000 BC. It continues to be one of the regular items of China's diet even today. Garlic was being grown in ancient China, Egypt, Greece and Rome and was used both as a staple food and a medicine for several ailments. It spread to all parts of the world and is now widely grown in India, Philippines, China, Ethiopia, Kenya, Brazil and Mexico.

## Food Value

Garlic has been held in high esteem for its health building qualities for centuries all over the world. Khnoum Khoufouf, the builder of one of the oldest pyramids, (4500 BC ) was among the first to recognise the true virtues of garlic for he decreed that all his workers should take garlic every day so that they could maintain their health and strength.

Hippocrates, the father of modern medicine (460-357 BC), who taught and practised in ancient Athens, recommended the use of this vegetable in infectious diseases and particularly prescribed it in intestinal disorders

An analysis of garlic shows it to contain high percentage of minerals and vitamins. It also contains traces of iodine, sulphur and chlorine.

## Garlic*

| Food Value | | Minerals and Vitamins | |
|---|---|---|---|
| Moisture | 62.0% | Calcium | 30 mg |
| Protein | 6.3% | Phosphorus | 310 mg |
| Fat | 0.1% | Iron | 1.3 mg |
| Minerals | 1.0% | Vitamin C | 13 mg |
| Fibre | 0.8% | Small amount of | |
| Carbohydrates | 29.8% | Vitamin B Complex | |
| | 100% | | |

*Values per 100 gms edible portion          **Calorific Value -** 145

## Natural Benefits and Curative Properties

In herbal medicine, garlic has been traditionally used for such ailments as asthma, deafness, leprosy, bronchial congestion, arteriosclerosis, fevers, worms and liver and gall bladder troubles. Babhet, an eminent Ayurvedic authority, is of the opinion that garlic is good for the heart, a food for the hair, a stimulant to appetite, a strengthening food, useful in leucoderma, leprosy, piles, worms, catarrhal disorders, asthma and cough

Clinical experiments in recent times have confirmed several ancient ideas about healing value of this vegetable. These experiments have in fact shown much greater power of garlic than known previously  The unpleasant odour in garlic, which constitutes its unpleasant feature and a serious social handicap, has been traced to its sulphur content. This mineral is contained to a greater degree in its volatile oil, which has marvellous therapeutic value. According to Dr. M.W. McDuffie of the Metropolitan Hospital, New York, "Garlic contains a volatile oil, called allyl sulphade, and its medical properties depend on this oil, strongly antiseptic, it seems to have a remarkable power of inhibiting the growth of the Koch's bacillus, eliminated by the lungs, skin, kidneys and liver, and oxidizes into sulphonic acid in the system. Applied locally, it is freely absorbed by the skin and penetrates the deeper tissues. Garlic gave us our best results, and would seem equally efficacious, no matter what part of the body affected, whether skin, bones, glands, lungs or special parts."[1]

---

1. Dr. S.J. Singh, *Food Remedies*, p. 89, Nature Cure Council of Medical Research, Lucknow, 1982.

Thus, garlic is regarded as a rejuvenetor. It has been found to help remove toxins, revitalise the blood, stimulate blood circulation and normalise intestinal flora. Garlic juice has a most beneficial effect on the entire system. The ethers in garlic juice are so potent and penetrating that they help to dissolve accumulation of mucus in the sinus cavities, in the bronchial tubes and in the lungs. They help the exudation of toxins from the body through the pores of the skin.

## Chest Diseases

Garlic has proved to be highly effective in certain diseases of the chest. It has been found to reduce fetidity of the breath in pulmonary gangrene. Dr. McDuffie advocated the use of garlic in tuberculosis of the lungs, Dr. F.W. Crosman once said that if garlic were given in sufficient quantities, it was a marvellous remedy in the treatment of pneumonia. This physician used garlic for many years in pneumonia, and said that in no instance did it fail to bring down the temperature, as well as the pulse and respiration, within 48 hours. Garlic can also be applied externally to the chest with beneficial results as it is an irritant and rubefacient.[2]

In *Ayurveda,* a decoction of garlic boiled in milk is considered a wonderful drug for tuberculosis. One gram of garlic, 240 ml of milk and 1 litre of water are boiled together till only one fourth of the decoction remains. It should be taken thrice in the day.

## Asthma

Three cloves of garlic boiled in milk, can be used every night with excellent results in asthma. A pod of garlic is peeled and macerated and boiled in 120ml. of pure malt-vinegar. After cooling it is strained and equal quantity of honey is mixed and preserved in a clean bottle. One or two teaspoons of this syrup taken with fenugreek decoction once in the evening and before retiring, has been found effective in reducing the severity of asthmatic attacks.[3]

## Digestive System Disorders

Garlic is one of the most beneficial foods for the digestive

2. Ibid. p. 87.

3 Dr. Aman, *Medicinal Secrets of Your Food,* p. 600 Indo-American Hospital, Mysore, 1985

system. It exercises a beneficial effect on the lymph, aids elimination of noxious waste matter in the body. It stimula peristaltic action and the secretion of the digestive juic Crushed cloves of garlic may be infused in water or milk and taken for all types of disorders of the digestion. It has an antiseptic effect and is an excellent remedy for infectious diseases and inflammations of the stomach and intestine. The oil of garlic is absorbed into the alimentary tract and is eliminated partly through the urine.

Garlic produces a very marked effects on the intestine. It is an excellent agent as a worm expeller. It has also a soothing effect on the various forms of diarrhoea. Problems such as colitis, dysentery and many other intestinal upsets can be successfully treated with fresh garlic or garlic capsules  One garlic capsule taken three times a day is usually sufficient to correct mild cases of diarrhoea or dysentery. For more persistent cases, upto six capsules a day can be taken. Garlic has the ability to destroy harmful bacteria in the intestines without affecting the beneficial organisms which aid digestion.

**High Blood Pressure**

Garlic is regarded as one of the most effective remedies to lower blood pressure. The pressure and tension are reduced because it has the power to ease the spasm of the small arteries. It also slows the pulse and modifies the heart rhythm, besides relieving the symptoms of dizziness, shortness of breath and the formation of gas within the digestive track  As these days garlic capsules are available with the chemist shops, the average dosage of two to three capsules a day to be given to make a dent in the blood pressure.

Dr. F.G Piotrowski, working at the University of Geneva, used garlic on 100 patients suffering from abnormally high blood pressure. In about 40 per cent of the cases treated, there was a significant reduction in blood pressure within one week of the treatment. Dr. Piotrowski claimed that garlic had a dilatory effect on the blood vessels, that is, it had the effect of making the blood vessels wider, thereby reducing the pressure.

**Rheumatic Affliction**

In Russia garlic is used extensively in the treatment of rheumatism and associated diseases. In Britain also garlic is recommended to rheumatic sufferers. Recent experiments in

Japan tested a garlic extract on patients with lumbago and arthritis and a large number of them were benefited without any undesirable side-effects Garlic has been shown to exhibit an anti-inflammatory property which could account for its effectiveness in the treatment of arthritis and rheumatism

The most popular method is to take the garlic cloves orally, although some reports indicate that pain can also be relieved by locally rubbing the affected parts with cloves of cut garlic. Garlic oil is rapidly absorbed through the skin and into the blood stream and quickly reaches the affected areas.

**Heart Attacks**

In a recent study, a West German doctor claims that garlic may prevent heart attacks. Professor Hams Reuter of Cologne University says that there is proof that garlic helps break up cholesterol in the blood vessels, thus helping in the prevention of hardening of arteries which leads to high blood pressure and heart attacks. If a patient takes garlic after a heart attack, the cholesterol level will come down. The earlier damage may not be repaired but its consumption will minimise the chances of new attacks.[4]

**Cancer**

Garlic preparations, including extracts and juices, have been used successfully against cancer in both animal and human studies, says Dr. Paavo Airola, a naturopathic physician and nutritionist A study report tells of mice being infected with cancer cells, some of which were then treated with garlic extract and some were not The mice not given garlic died within 16 days the other mice lived for six months. And recent studies done in Russia have found garlic preparations to retard tumour growth not only in animals, but also in human beings, writes Dr. Airola [5]

**Skin Disorders**

Garlic has also been used successfully for a variety of skin disorders Pimples disappear without scar when rubbed with raw garlic several times a day. Even very persistent form of acne, suffered by some adults, has also been healed with garlic. The

---

4 M.K Kaul *Mirror*, Monthly Magazine, Bombay, p. 40, June 1986 issue
5 Ibid

118

external use of garlic helps to clear the skin of spots and pimples and boils. The process is further helped by taking the garlic orally also, to purify the blood-steam so as to secure a long-term clearance of the skin. A regular course of three garlic capsules per day should help to clear minor skin infections quickly.

## Wounds and Ulcers

Garlic has been used as an antiseptic in wounds and ulcerations with beneficial results. Garlic juice with three parts of distilled water has been employed as a lotion for cleansing infected wounds. Definite improvement is noticed within 24 hours and substantial improvement within 48 hours.[6] Application of dressing containing 15 per cent garlic juice once a day over an ulcer removes pus in a few days. It also relieves pain within a short time. Russian physicians are making extensive use of garlic in the healing of wounds.

## Diphtheria

Garlic is considered an excellent remedy for diphtheria. Its constant application by chewing a clove of garlic removes the membranes, reduces temperature and relieves the patient. About 30 or 60 gms. of garlic can be used in this way in three or four hours for a week  After the membrane disappears, the same quantity of garlic should be chewed daily. The diphtheric patient has no taste or smell and merely finds the garlic hot.[7]

## Whooping Cough

Garlic is an excellent remedy for whooping cough. Syrup of garlic should be given in doses of five drops to a teaspoonful two or three times a day in this condition. It should be given more often if the coughing spells are frequent and violent.[8]

## Sexual Debility

Garlic is a natural and harmless aphrodisiac. Even Dr. Robinson, an eminent sexologist of America considers it so. It is a tonic for loss of sexual power from any cause, sexual debility, impotency from over indulgence in sex and nervous exhaustion from dissipating habit. It is said to be especially useful to old

---

6. Col. R.N Chopra, *Indigenous Drugs of India*, p. 273. Academic Publishers, Calcutta, 1982.

7. Ibid.

8. Dr. S.J. Singh, *Food Remedies*, p 91, Nature Cure Council of Medical Research, Lucknow, 1982.

men of high nervous tension and diminishing sexual power.[9]

**Uses**

Garlic like onions, leeks, and various garden flower belongs to the plant of genus called Allium. Garlic is the most widely used of the cultivated alliums after onions. It is used both as a food and seasoning. It is, however, extensively used as flavouring and seasoning in the preparation of soups, sauces and pickles. In Spain and Italy it is used in combination with almost every food.

# *Ginger*

Botanical Name : *Zingiber officinalse*
Indian Name : *Adrak*

**Description**

Ginger is a perennial herb, with underground branching stems called rhizomes which are swollen and tough. They are white or yellow outside and become grey-brown or orange with age, upto 2.5 cm in diameter. Leaves and rhizomes have characteristic fragrant odour when cut or bruised. Rhizomes are dug out after the leafy parts are dried. They are sold as fresh ginger in the vegetable market or are peeled, sliced and dried. The sun-dried ginger is commonly known as *sount* in India.

**Origin and Distribution**

Ginger is believed to have originated in India and was introduced in China at a very early date. It appears to have been used as a spice and a medicine from early times by the Indians and the Chinese. There are numerous references to it in Sanskrit literature and in Chinese Medical treatises. It was known in Europe in first century AD and was mentioned by Dioscorides and Pliny As living rhizomes of ginger are very easy to transport, the plant soon spread to all tropical countries. The sanskrit name *singebera* gave rise to the Greek *Zingiberi* and to the late latin *Zingiber*. The major producers today are China, India and Taiwan.

---

9  Ibid, p, 92

Ginger is cultivated all over India, but ginger grown in Kerala is found to be superior than the ones grown in other places, in aroma and in taste.

**Food Value**

Ginger is available in two forms, fresh and dried. Both the forms contain effective food value. As the taste of ginger is not very palatable, subtle means are adopted to use it in certain ways. It is put in vegetables. The dried ginger, which may be scraped or peeled before drying, constitute the spice, and is esteemed for its flavour, pungency, aroma and medicinal value.

### Ginger*

| Food Value | | Minerals and Vitamins | |
|---|---|---|---|
| Moisture | ·80.9% | Calcium | 20 mg |
| Protein | 2.3% | Phosphorus | 60 mg |
| Fat | 0.9% | Iron | 2.6 mg |
| Minerals | 1.2% | Vitamin C | 6 mg |
| Fibre | 2.4% | Small amount of | |
| Carbohydrates | 12.3% | Vitamin B Complex | |
| | 100% | | |
| *Values per 100 gms edible portion | | **Calorific Value - 67** | |

**Natural Benefits and Curative Properties**

Ginger is being used as medicine in India from Vedic period and is called *Maha-aushidhi,* meaning the great medicine. Ancient physicians used ginger as a carminative and anti fermenting medicine. Galen, the Greek physician, used ginger as a medicine to rectify the defective humours of the body. He used ginger in the treatment of paralysis caused by phlegmatic imbalance in the body. Aviceena, another Greek physician used it as an aphrodisiac. Pomose, yet another Greek physician also used ginger in the treatment of gout centuries ago.[1]

Ginger is now widely used in local medicines in India and the far East. Taken internally, it is a stimulating carminative and locally it is used as a rubefacient and counter-irritant. Like many other spices, ginger is believed to have aphrodisiac properties.

The ginger yields an essential oil, but this lacks the pungent

---

1. Dr. Aman, *Medicinal Secrets of Your Food,* p. 606, Indo-American Hospital, Mysore, 1985.

principle, it is used in the manufacture of flavouring essence and in perfumery An oleoresin — i.e. mixture of oil and resin — is also extracted, in which the full pungency of the spice is preserved; it is used for flavouring and also for medicinal purposes.

## Digestive System Disorders

Ginger is a valuable drug for disorders of the digestive system. It is extremely useful in dyspepsia, flatulence, colic, vomiting, spasms and other painful affections of the stomach and the bowels. Chewing a piece of fresh ginger after meals regularly is an insurance against these ailmets. This protective action is attributable to excessive secretion of saliva, diastate enzyme and volatile oil.

Half a teaspoon of fresh ginger juice, mixed with one teaspoonful of each of fresh lime juice and fresh mint juice and a tablespoonful of honey, constitutes an effective medicine for dyspepsia, nausea and vomiting due to a biliousness, indigestion caused by intake of heavy non-vegetarian and fried fatty food, morning sickness, jaundice and piles. This mixture should be sucked thrice daily in the treatment of these conditions.[2]

## Cough and Cold

Ginger is an excellent remedy for coughs and colds. Extracted juice of ginger with honey should be taken three or four times a day in case of coughs. In case of colds, ginger should be cut into small pieces and boiled in a cup of water. It should then be strained and half a teaspoon of sugar added to it It should be drunk while hot. Ginger tea, prepared by adding few pieces of ginger into boiled water before adding tea leaves, is also an effective remedy for colds and for fevers resulting from cold

## Respiratory Disorders

A teaspoonful of the fresh ginger juice mixed with a cupful of fenugreek decoction and honey to taste is an excellent diaphoretic mixture which increases sweating to reduce fever in influenza. It acts as an expectorant in bronchitis, asthma, whooping cough and tuberculosis of the lungs.[3]

---

2. Ibid., p. 607.
3. Ibid., p. 608.

**Aches and Pains**

Ginger is an excellent pain killer. It can cure all types of pain. In headache, ginger ointment made by rubbing dry ginger with a little water and applied to the forehead affords relief. It allays tooth ache when applied to the face. In case of earache, a few drops of ginger juice will give relief.

**Sexual Debility**

Ginger juice is a valuable aphrodisiac. It is highly beneficial in the treatment of sexual weakness For better results, half a teaspoon of ginger juice should be taken with a half-boiled egg and honey, once, daily at night for a month. It tones up the sex centres and cures impotency, premature ejaculation, spermatorrhoea.

**Menstrual Disorders**

Ginger is also useful in menstrual disorders. A piece of fresh ginger should be pounded and boiled in a cupful of water for few minutes. The infusion sweetened with sugar should be taken thrice daily after meals as a medicine for dysmenorrhoea, and amenorrhoea due to exposure to cold winds and taking cold bath.[4]

**Uses**

In western countries, it is widely used for culinary purposes in gingerbread, biscuits, cakes, puddings, soups and pickles. But it is used as curry powder all over the world. Ginger is the most widely-used spice in Chinese cookery It is used in the production of ginger beer, ginger ale and ginger wine. It was formerly much used for spicing wines, possets and porter, the last one often being stirred with a red-hot poker.

# *Lettuce*

Botanical Name *Lactuca sativa*
Indian Name *Kahu or Kasmi-sāg, Salād pattā*

**Description**

Lettuce is regarded as the king of salad plants. It is most

---

4. Hakeem Mahamood Shariff, *Zathi Tajrubath*, Urdu MS Chamraj Nagar, 1968.

popular of all the salad vegetables  It has rounded leaves upto 25 cms. in length and 15 cms. in width. Leaves and stem contain milky juice. There are several varieties of lettuce. They differ in colour of the leaves, size and texture. The colour of leaves varies from light to dark green. Broadly two varieties are generally used at table, namely, the loose-leaf lettuce and the true head-lettuce In the loose-leaf lettuce the leaves hang on all side. The head lettuce is like a cabbage with the leaves drawn together

## Origin and Distribution

The centre of origin of lettuce appears to be the Middle-East. The first records of lettuce as a vegetable in a long-leaved form are depicted on Egyptian tombs dated 4500 BC. It was used by the Persian royalty more than 550 years before Christ. Lettuce was cultivated as a salad plant by the ancient Greeks and Romans

Lettuce reached China in the seventh century AD. It was first used in England in 1520 and King Henry VIII is said to have conferred a special reward upon the gardener who devised the combination of lettuce and cherries for the royal table. Lettuce is comparatively a recent introduction into the tropics. It is now widely cultivated in India, Malaysia, Indonesia, the Philippines, China, the Caribbean, Central and South America and East, West and Central Africa

## Food Value

Lettuce is a live food with its rich vitamin content, especially the antiscorbutic vitamin C. It is bulky, low in food value but high in health value. It is rich in mineral salts with the alkaline elements greatly predominating. So it helps to keep the blood clean, the mind alert and body in good health.

### Lettuce*

| Food Value | | Minerals and Vitamins | |
|---|---|---|---|
| Moisture | 93.4% | Calcium | 50 mg |
| Protein | 2.1% | Phosphorus | 28 mg |
| Fat | 0.3% | Iron | 2.4 mg |
| Minerals | 1.2% | Vitamin C | 10 mg |
| Fibre | 0.5% | Small amount of | |
| Carbohydrates | 2.5% | Vitamin B Complex | |
| | 100% | | |

*Values per 100 gms edible portion          **Calorific Value – 42**

The loose-leaf lettuce is considered a better food. It has the advantage of being more exposed to sunlight, thus providing it with a richer supply of vitamins than the head-lettuce in which the leaves are closed. Whatever qualitty of lettuce is selected for use, it should be ensured that it is fresh, crisp and green — leaved. The greener the leaves, the higher the vitamins.

## Natural Benefits and Curative Properties

Lettuce contains several health-building qualities and many medicinal virtues. It has many essential values to the human body. It is very good for brain, nervous system and lungs. The raw juice of lettuce is cool and refreshing. The high content of magnesium in the juice has exceptional power to vitalise the muscular tissues, the nerves and the brain.

When making juice from lettuce for definite therapeutic purposes, it is best to use the leaves that are of the darker shade of green. The leaves which are inside the head of lettuce and have remained white should be discared. The former are much richer in chlorophyll and other vital elements than the latter.

### Constipation

As lettuce is rich in cellulose, it increases the bulk of the intestinal contents and encourages peristalsis. It is, therefore, highly beneficial in curing chronic constipation.

### Insomnia

Lettuce is beneficial in the treatment of insomnia as it contains a sleep inducing substance. called "lectucarium". Lettuce juice has been likened in effect to the sedative action of opium without the accompanying excitement. According to Culpepper, the ancient English herbalist, the juice of lettuce mixed with oil of roses, applied to the forehead and temples, induces sleep and eases the head-ache.[1] The seeds of lettuce in decoction are useful in insomnia and wakefulness due to mental overwork.

### Diabetes

Lettuce belongs to that group of vegetables which contain three per cent or less of carbohydrate. It is, therefore, among the important foods which can be prescribed for diabetes. It can be used freely by diabetics

---

1. Susane E. Charmaine, *The Complete Raw Juice Therapy*, p. 78 Thorsons Publishing Group, Great Britain, 1987.

## Anaemia

Lettuce contains considerable amount of iron and supplies a good form of vegetable haemoglobin. It can, therefore, be used as a good tonic food for anaemia. The iron obtained in this way is absorbed by the body to a much greater degree than the inorganic iron tonic

## Pregnancy and Lactation

Eating raw lettuce has a highly beneficial effect during pregnancy and lactation. A very important nutritional factor, folic acid, contained in lettuce prevents megaloblastic anaemia during pregnancy. In a series of experiments with lettuce, its useful effect during pregnancy confirms that mothers who had a regular use of lettuce were free from nutritional anaemia. One particular benefit of lettuce eating is that it prevents habitual abortions. It is believed to have a great influence over the secretion of progesterone hormone. Eating lettuce with spinach, peas, asparagus and cauliflower increases the folic acid or vitamin B content of the food. It is estimated that about 300-500 mcg. of this vitamin is daily required during the last trimester of pregnancy.[2] The deficiency of which causes magaloblastic anaemia.

## Uses

Lettuce is normally used in the raw state as salad. The leaves are also cooked as greens, especially loose-leaf lettuce. It will cook in almost no water at all. The water which clings after washing will suffice. It should be kept covered over a stove for the first few minutes until the juice starts flowing. It should then be cooked uncovered for about 10 minutes.

## Precautions

Lettuce leaves should be washed thoroughly before use as salad. They should be washed leaf by leaf. When thoroughly clean, they should be put repeatedly within the folds of a clean towel until the leaves are completely dry

2. Dr. Aman, *Medicinal Secrets of Your Food*, p. 360, Indo-American Hospital, Mysore, 1985

# *Mint*

Botanical Name : *Minthe spicata*
Indian Name : *Pudina*

### Description

Mint is a popular spice, used extensively in Indian cooking. It is an erect, branched perennial herb with underground modified stems. The Shoots produced from these stems are four-angled, and bear oval-shaped leaves which are simple, delicate, thin, dark green in colour and fragrant.

### Origin and Distribution

Mint is a native of temperate Europe. Ancient Romans and Greeks knew about this plant. In olden days it was believed that Minthe, the damsel lover of God Pulto, was transferred into this herb due to the anger of Persephone, the wife of Pulto and Goddess of Wealth. Therefore mint is commonly known as Minthae in Latin. The ancient Greek physician, Saufarsats used mint in the preparation of various carminative medicines. Even Mohammadan physicians were familiar with this herb. Chinese and Japanese knew this herb as long as two thousand years.[1] Mint has now been introduced in all parts of the world and it widely grows in Indonesia, West Africa etc. In India, mint grows widely in Himalayan plains and Kashmir valley in a number of varieties.

### Food Value

**Mint***

| Food Value | | Minerals and Vitamins | |
|---|---|---|---|
| Moisture | 84.9% | Calcium | 200 mg |
| Protein | 4.8% | Phosphorus | 62 mg |
| Fat | 0.6% | Iron | 15.6 mg |
| Minerals | 1.9% | Vitamin C | 27 mg |
| Fibre | 2.0% | Small amounts of | |
| Carbohydrates | 5.8% | Vitamin B Complex | |
| | 100% | and good amount of | |
| | | Vitamin D and E | |
| *Value per 100 gms edible portion | | **Calorific Value - 48** | |

1. Dr. Aman, *Medicinal Secrets of Your Food*, p. 363, Indo American Hospital, Mysore, 1985.

Mint contains plenty of vitamins and is rich in several minerals. The fresh and dried leaves are used for mint sauce and jelly and to flavour foods. Mint oil is used in chewing gum, tooth paste and in confectionery and pharmaceutical preparations.

## Natural Benefits and Curative Properties

Mint is much valued as a carminative which relieves gastric discomforts, stimulant, antispasmodic which relieves muscle strain and stomachic for improving appetite. It forms an ingredient of most drugs prescribed for stomach ailments because of its digestive properties It is good for the liver and helps dissolve gravel in the kidneys and bladder.

### Digestive System Disorders

Mint juice is a good appetiser. Fresh leaf juice of mint mixed with a teaspoonful of lime juice and honey is given thrice daily with excellent results in the treatment of indigestion, biliousness, flatulent colic, thread worms, morning sickness and summer diarrhoea.

According to father Kneipp, the well-known Naturopath, "A cupful of mint tea taken every morning and evening assists the digestion and gives a fresh and healthy appearance. The powder renders the same service, if one or two pinches are taken daily in the food or in water." He also considers that mint, prepared in milk or tea and drunk warm, removes abdominal pains.[2]

The seeds of mint are also beneficial in relieving severe abdominal pain due to indigestion in older children. The child may be given a quarter teaspoonful of the seeds to chew and swallow with water in such conditions

### Respiratory Disorders

A teaspoonful of fresh mint juice, mixed with two spoonfuls of pure malt vinegar and equal quantity of honey is stirred in four ounces of carrot juice and is given thrice daily as a medicated tonic during the treatment of tuberculosis, asthma and bronchitis. It liquifies the sputum, nourishes the lungs, increases body's resistance against infection and prevents the harmful effects of anti tubercular drugs It prevents the asthmatic attacks and reduces congestion in air passages.

---

2. Dr. S.J. Singh, *Food Remedies,* p. 142, Nature Cure Council of Medical Research, Lucknow, 1982.

## Oral Disorders

Fresh leaves of mint, chewed daily is an effective antiseptic dentifrice i.e. tooth paste. The chlorophyll combined with other antiseptic chemicals in the mint, kills all the germs causing harmful odour. It strengthens the gums by providing the required nutrients and thus prevents tooth decay, pyorrhoea, pre-mature fall of the teeth etc. It also keeps the mouth fresh and improves the sense of taste in the tongue.

## Hoarseness

Gargling fresh mint decoction with salt cures hoarseness due to shouting or singing loudly. It keeps the voice clear if used before singing. Therefore, it is a boon to singers and orators.[3]

## Skin Disorders

Application of fresh mint juice over face every night, cures pimples and prevents dryness of the skin. Juice is also applied over insect stings, eczema, scabies and contact dermatitis.

## Natural Birth-Control

In *Ayurveda,* powdered dry mint is regarded as a harmless herb for birth control. It is believed that the woman who swallows 10 grams of this powder a little before the sexual intercourse will be free from pregnancy so long as she continues this practice. The mint should be dried in a shady place and then powdered and bottled.[4]

# Onion

Botanical Name : *Allium cepa*
Indian Name : *Piyāz*

## Description

The onion, a pungent edible of the lily family, is one of the oldest cultivated vegetables. It is considered a food of exceptional value for flavouring and seasoning.

---

3. Ibid, p. 369.
4. Kvj. Ganpati Singh Verma, *Miracles of Indian Herbism,* p. 115, Rasayan Pharmacy, New Delhi, 1982.

The onion is a biennial herb, usually grown as an annual. All its parts produce a strong onion odour when crushed. It has superficial root system, a very short flattened stem at the base of the plant, which increases in diametre as growth continues. Leaves are long, linear and hollow. A bulb is formed by thickening of the leaf bases when the plant reaches a certain stage of growth. The fruit is a globular capsule.

## Origin and Cultivation

Onion is believed to have originated in Central Asia, possibly in the Iran-Pakistan region. It has been cultivated since ancient times in the Middle East and India. It was a popular food in ancient Egypt, where it is depicted on tombs as early as 3200 BC and has been found in mummies.

The Sanskrit equivalent for onion is *palandu* which has been mentioned in the *Garuda Purana*. The great Indian sages, Maharishi Atreya and Lord Dhanwantri have described the use of onions in details. It is referred to in the *Bible*, when the Israelites complained of their hardships while being led by Moses from Egypt to the land of Canaan about 1500 BC remembering the onions that they ate in Egypt.

Onion is frequently referred to in the literature from Hippocrates, 430 BC down to the present time. It is on record that the Jews loved onions so much that they named a city after it —Onion. This city was built in 173 BC near the Gulf of Suez. The man who built it was called Onions. The city existed for 343 years.

Onion is now cultivated in most parts of the world, including India, Malaysia, Indonesia, Burma, Philippines, China, Egypt, West and East Africa, tropical South and Central America and the Caribbean.

## Food Value

Onion which derived its name from the Latin *Onio* and French *Oignon,* has been described by some one as the dynamite of natural foods. Compared with other fresh vegetables, it is relatively high in food value, moderate in protein content and is rich in calcium and riboflavin. There is considerable variation in composition between different varieties and it also varies with the stage of maturity and the length of storage.

The odour in onion is due to organic sulphur compounds, and is produced only when the tissues are cut or injured, by

| Food Value | | Minerals and Vitamins | |
|---|---|---|---|
| Moisture | 86.6% | Calcium | 47 mg |
| Protein | 1.2% | Phosphorus | 50 mg |
| Fat | 0.1% | Iron | 0.7 mg |
| Fibre | 0.6% | Vitamin C | 11 mg |
| Minerals | 0.4% | Small amount of | |
| Carbohydrates | 11.1% | Vitamin B Complex | |
| | 100% | | |
| *Values 100 gms edible portion | | **Calorific Value - 51** | |

enzyme action on a water-soluble amino acid. Heating, freezing and drying prevent the enzyme action. That is why cooking produces a different odour, flavour and pungency. The pungent flavour of onion is much appreciated by many people in many countries. The strong odour lingers for a considerable time after consumption. It is said to be due to small particles retained in the mouth which cannot always be removed by brushing.

The onion has a good keeping quality. The dried cured bulbs may be kept for several months without deterioration and can stand rough handling. Good storage life is usually associated with high pungency

## Natural Benefits and Curative Properties

Onion is highly valued for its therapeutic properties. It has been used as a food remedy from time immemorial The physicians of ancient Egypt prescribed onions in various diseases. Dioscorides in the first century AD attributed many herbal remedies to them. They are stimulent, diuretic, expectorant and rubefacient

The white onion is preferable to the red and yellow varieties. Onions should be taken with meals preferably raw as fried or cooked onions are comparatively difficult to digest. For therapeutic purposes, it is advisable to use onion juice instead of the whole onion as it is an alround medicine. Onion being stimulating and irritating food, its consumption in excess should be avoided.

Several parts of the plant have a place in the traditional medicines. The seeds of onion increase semen and relieve dental worms and urinary diseases. The stalks of onion are a source of Vitamin A, thiamin and ascorbic acid They are used in both tender and mature stages.

## Respiratory Disease

Onion is said to possess expectorant properties. It liquifies phelgm and prevents its further formation. It has been used as a food remedy for centuries in cold, cough, bronchitis and influenza. Equal amounts of onion juice and honey should be mixed and three to four teaspoon of this mixture should be taken daily in these conditons. It is one of the safest preventive medicine against common cold during winter.

## Tooth Disorders

Latest researches of Russian doctors have further confirmed the bactericidal properties of onion. According to these findings, if a person consumes one raw onion every day by thorough mastication, he will be protected from a host of tooth disorders. The Russian Doctor, B.P. Tohkin, who has contributed to this research, has expressed the opinion that chewing raw onion for three minutes is sufficient to kill all the germs in the mouth. Toothache is often allayed by placing a small piece of onion on the bad tooth or gum.

## Anaemia

Onions are noted for their easily assimilable iron content. They are, therefore, beneficial in the treatment of anaemia.

## Heart Disease

Recent researches in the West have established onion as an effective preventive food item against heart-attack. Dr. N.N. Gupta of the K.G. Medical College, Lucknow, in 1966, and a panel of doctors in England in 1968 have stated that onion has been found helpful and beneficial in diseases of the heart. According to them these benefits are due to the presence of essential oil, aliypropyl disulphide, catechol, protocatechnic acid, thiopropiono aldehyde, thiocyanate, calcium, iron, phosphorus and vitamins in onion.

Dr. N. Radhakrishnan, Principal of the Trivandrum Medical College and Dr. K. Madhavan Kutty have established, after seven years of research, that to get rid of coronary heart or blood pressure disorders and one should take 100 gms. of onion per day. The onion are very valuable in heart diseases as they correct thrombosis and also reduce blood cholesterol.[1]

---

1. Dr. S.J. Singh, *Food Remedies* p. 146 *Nature Cure Council* of Medical Research, Lucknow, 1982.

## Sexual Debility

Onion is one of the most important aphrodisiac foods. As an aphrodisiac, onion stands second only to garlic. It increases libido and strengthens the reproductory organs. The white variety of onion should be peeled off, crushed and fried in pure butter. This mixture acts as an excellent aphrodisiac tonic if taken regularly with a spoon of honey on an empty stomach. The powder of black gram when diped in the juice of onion for seven days and then dried, produces a mixture called *kanji*. This also acts an an aphrodisiac.[2]

## Skin Disorders

Onion is irritating to the skin and stimulates the circulation of blood in the mucous membrane. Warts also sometimes disappear if rubbed with cut onions. Roasted or otherwise, onions are applied as a poultice to boils, bruises, wounds, etc., to bring the boils to-maturity by its heaty sensation.

## Ear Disorders

Onion juice dipped on cotton wool and put into the ear is a popular Russian remedy for ringing sound in the ears. Dropped hot in the ear, it relieves earache.

## Cholera

Onion is an effective remedy for cholera. About 30 grams of onion and seven black peppers should be finely pounded in a pestle and given to the patient of cholera. It allays thirst and restlessness and the patient feels better. It also lessens vomiting and diarrhoea immediately. An addition to little sugar to the recipe will increase its effectivenes.[3]

## Urinary System Disorders

Onions are highly beneficial in the treatment of urinary system disorders. For burning sensation in urine, six grams of onion should be boiled in 500 ml. of water. It should be removed from the fire when half the water has evaporated. It should then be strained, allowed to cool and given to the patient as a drink. It will relieve the burning sensation in urine. Onion rubbed in water and mixed with 60 grams of sugar will be useful in retention of urine. It will bring about free urination within a

---

2. "Treatment by Orions for Cure and Prevention of Disease", Prakritrani, Monthly Magazine, January, 1988. p. 9.

3. Ibid., p. 10.

short time.[4]

**Bleeding Piles**

Onions are valuable in bleeding piles. About 30 grams of onions should be finely rubbed in water and 60 grams or sugar added to it. It should be taken twice daily by the patient. It will bring relief within a few days.

**Uses**

The onion can be used in innumerable ways. The immature and mature bulbs are eaten raw or they may be cooked and eaten as a vegetable. They are used in soups and sauces and for seasoning many foods. They may also be fried. Coated with gram flour and fried, the onion *bhajiya* makes an excellent snack. Small white leaf at the base before the bulb are eaten raw in salads. These immature plants are known as green, bunching or spring onions. Onion oil, produced by steam distillation, is used to a limited extent for flavouring foods.

There has been an increasing demand, in recent years, for dehydrated onion products. The onions are sliced and dried. They are used for flavouring food and in canned meat products, sausages, canned and dried soups and ketchups. Dried onion flakes can be reconstituted by cooking in water, and are used in salads and other foods. Chopped and dried green onion tops may be used as a substitute for chives—a kind culinary herb for culinary purposes.

# *Potato*

Botanical Name : *Solanum tuberosum*
Indian Name : *Alu*

**Description**

The potato is the most popular and widely used vegetable in the world. It is an annual plant, producing swollen underground stem tubers. This vegetable forms an indispensable item of daily food and is an important source of nutrition.

4. Kvj. Ganpati Singh Verma, *Miracles of Onions*, p. 16. Rasayan Pharmacy, Delhi, 1981.

**Origin and Distribution**

The potato is a native of South America, where it has been cultivated from ancient times. It was introduced to Europe in the later-half of the 16th century. But nearly one hundred years, it was looked upon as a poisonous tuber. Its food value was realised only in 1771, when a prize was offered in France for the discovery of an article of food which could be used as substitute for wheat in times of famine.

In the United States, potato was introduced by Irish immigrants in 1719. The Spaniards took it to Philippines at an early date. It came to India in the 17th century. The missionaries probably introduced it into East Africa towards the end of the 19th century. In volume and value a world basis, the potato now exceeds all other crops in the world.

**Food Value**

Potato contains high nutritive value. Its chief food principle is starch, but it has a notable amount of protein of high biological value. It contains a substantial amount of alkaline salts. It is rich in soda, potash and vitamins A and B.

**Potato***

| Food Value | | Minerals and Vitamins | |
|---|---|---|---|
| Moisture | 74.7% | Calcium | 10 mg |
| Protein | 1.6% | Phosphorus | 40 mg |
| Fat | 0.1% | Iron | 0.7 mg |
| Minerals | 0.6% | Vitamin C | 17 mg |
| Fibre | 0.4% | Small amount of | |
| Carbohydrates | 22.6% | Vitamin B Complex | |
| | 100% | | |
| *Values per 100 gms edible portion | | **Calorific Value - 97** | |

The potato can be boiled, baked. steamed and cooked with other vegetables. But it should be cooked in such a way so as to retain all its excellent qualities. To secure its maximum value, it should always be cooked with its skin as the most nutritive part of the potato lies just below the skin and this particular layer is very rich in protein and mineral salts.

## Natural Benefits and Curative Properties

The potato contains several medicinal virtues. As it is one of the most strongly alkaline of all foods, it is, therefore, very helpful in maintaining the alkali reserve of the body and a natural antidote for an overdose of acid or acidosis. It dissolves away uric acid and lime. It is also important in preventing the fermentative process in intestine and it helps the growth of friendly bacteria in the digestive tract.

However, potatoes should be avoided by obese people as they are fattening. They should also be omitted from the diet of those suffering from venereal diseases and those afflicted with aphrodisiac tendencies. The potato contains an alkaloid toxin known as solanine which affects the nerves controlling the sexual organs. The solanine poison is particularly prevalent in potatoes too green in colour. The combination of cooked meat and potatoes too green in colour. The combination of cooked meat and potatoes intensifies the solanine poison, which together with presence of uric acid crystals resulting from the ingestion of meat may cause excessive irritation of sexual organs.

**Potato Therapy**

An exclusive potato diet is considered valuable in the treatment of certain disorders such as chronic constipation, intestinal toxaemia, uric acid diseases, renal calculi or stone and dropsy. This diet may be employed with beneficial results for several months, if necessary. In the potato diet, potatoes can be consumed in its various preparations, such as baked, steamed and in soup form. When on potato diet, other vegetables which can be taken are spinach, beet tops, turnip tops, cucumbers lettuce, celery, tomatoes and other green vegetables.

**Scurvy**

The potato is regarded as an excellent food remedy in scurvy. It has been noted that scurvy in Europe has become more and more uncommon with the progress of potato cultivation and it makes its appearance only when the crop fails. Dr. G.F. Still used "potato cream" in curing cases of infantile scurvy, while Dr. A.F. Hess used ordinary mashed potatoes for the same purposes.[1]

**Rheumatism**

Raw potato juice is regarded as an excellent food remedy for

1. Dr. S.J. Singh, *Food Remedies*, p. 174, Nature Cure Council of Medical Research, Lucknow, 1982.

rheumatism. One or two teaspoonful of the juice pressed out of mashed raw potato should be taken before meals. This will help eliminate an acid condition and relieve rheumatism. In some rural areas in Great Britain, it is a custom for rheumatic sufferer to carry a potato in their pockets, in the belief that the potato will absorb in itself some of the acid from the sufferer's body. The old potato is thrown away and replaced by new one after a few days.

The skin of the potato is also an excellent food remedy for rheumatism. The skin is exceptionally rich in vital mineral salts and the water in which the peelings have been boiled is one of the best medicines for the ailments caused by excess of acid in the system. The potato peelings should be thoroughly washed and boiled for few minutes. The decoction should then by strained and a glassful of the same should be taken three or four times daily.[2]

### Digestive System Disorders

Raw potato juice is valuable in stomach and intestinal disorders. Stomach ulcers are treated with the juice of pink potatoes. Potato juice also relieves gastritis. The recommended dose is half a cupful two or three times half an hour before meals. Potato starch is administered as an anti-inflammatory for gastro-intestinal diseases and toxins.

### Skin Blemishes

The juice of raw potatoes, has also proved very valuable in clearing skin blemishes. This cleansing results from high content of potassium, sulphur, phosphorus and chlorine in the potato. These elements are, however, of value only when the potato is raw as in this state they are composed of live organic atoms. In the cooked state, they are converted into inorganic atoms and are of little value for constructive purposes.[3]

The juicy pulp of the shredded raw potatoes can also be applied as a poultice in clearing the wrinkles and other skin blemishes due to ageing. It may be rubbed on the face and other portions of body that have wrinkles before retiring for bed. It will help 'melt' the wrinkles, banish age spots and clear the skin.

---

2. Eric F.W. Powell, *Health from The Kitchen*, p. 20, Health Science Press, England, 1973.

3. N.W. Walker, *Raw Vegetable Juices*. p. 77, Jove Books. New York, 1983.

The enzymes in raw potato pulp, combined with the Vitamin C and the natural starch, helps create a 'skin food' that nourishes the starved cellular tissues of the skin. Furthermore, the alkaline juices of the potato promotes an antiseptic action that gives a glowing look of youth. Much of the decaying skin sloughs off by the acid portion of the pulp[4].

## Swellings

Raw potato juice, externally applied, is valuable in the treatment of swelling and other disordered condition of the joints and muscles. After extraction of the juice, it should be boiled down to about one-fifth of its original bulk. A little quantity of glycerine may be added as a preservative. It is used as liniment. It should be applied after fomentation of the affected parts and should be repeated every three hours until the pain and swelling are relieved.

# *Radish*

Botanical Name : *Raphanus sativus*

Indian Name : *Muli*

## Description

The radish is one of the most commonly used vegetables in India. It is an hairy annual herb. It has no stem or branches. it has only one root which is round, cylindrical or tapering, white or red, slightly coarse, fleshy, succulent, and 3 to 7 cm thick, 10 to 20 cm long. It has a pungent flavour. It stimulates appetite and promotes a healthy bloodstream.

There are many varieties of radish, differing in size and colour. The red and white coloured are most familiar. They are tender when young but become woody and tough as they mature.

## Origin and Distribution

Radish is believed to have originated in Western Asia. It was

---

4. Carlson Wade, *Health Secrets from the Orient*, p. 65, Allied Publishers Pvt. Ltd., Delhi.

cultivated in ancient Egypt, Greece and Rome. It has now spread all over the world. Its areas of cultivation include South America. East and West Africa, the Caribbean, Malaysia, Indonesia, India, China and most tropical areas.

**Food Value**

The radish is one of the richest sources of iron, calcium and sodium of all the common vegetables. The roots, rather than the leaves of these small plants, are generally used as food item. They should be eaten raw to derive all its beneficial effects. Cooking destroys its vitamin content and thus cooked vegetable looses its powerful antiscorbutic properties. However, the leaves are also eaten as salad or used in cooking. Radish leaves have more calcium, phosphorus, Vitamin C and protein than radish itself.

### Radish*

| Food Value | | Minerals and Vitamins | |
|---|---|---|---|
| Moisture | 94.4% | Calcium | 35 mg |
| Protein | 0.7% | Phosphorus | 22 mg |
| Fat | 0.1% | Iron | 0.4 mg |
| Minerals | 0.6% | Vitamin C | 15 mg |
| Fibre | 0.8% | Small amount of | |
| Carbohydrates | 3.4% | Vitamin B Complex | |
| | 100% | | |

Calorific Value - 17

### Radish Leaves*

| Food Value | | Minerals and Vitamins | |
|---|---|---|---|
| Moisture | 90.8% | Calcium | 265 mg |
| Protein | 3.8% | Phosphorus | 59 mg |
| Fat | 0.4% | Iron | 3.6 mg |
| Minerals | 1.6% | Vitamin C | 81 mg |
| Fibre | 1.0% | Small amount of | |
| Carbohydrates | 2.4% | Vitamin B Complex | |
| | 100% | | |

*Values per 100 gms edible portion          Calorific Value - 28

## Natural Benefits and Curative Properties

The leaves of radish are diuretic, antiscorbutic and laxative. The tap root is also strongly antiscorbutic for preventing of curing scurvy and the seeds are expectorant, diuretic, carminative for relieving gastric discomforts, laxative and stimulant.

## Piles

The juice and the fresh root is regarded as an effective food remedy in piles. It should be given in doses of 60 to 90 ml. morning and evening.

## Genito-Urinary Disorders

This juice is also beneficial in the treatment of dysuria on painful urination and stranguary or severe urethral pain. It may be given in doses mentioned above and repeated as often as necessary. A cupful of radish leaf-juice given once daily for a fortnight acts as a curative medicine in dissolving gravel in urinary tract and cystitis—i.e. inflammation of urinary bladder.

## Chest Complaints

A syrup prepared by mixing a teaspoonful of fresh radish juice with equal quantity of honey and a little rock salt is highly beneficial in the treatment of hoarseness, whooping cough, bronchial disorders and other chest complaints. It should be given thrice daily.

## Jaundice

Green leaves of radish are beneficial in the treatment of jaundice. The leaves should be pounded and their juice expressed out through a piece of thin cloth. It should be sweetened to one's taste by adding fine crystaline sugar. About half a Kg. of this juice should be taken daily by an adult patient. This provides immediate relief. The preparation induces healthy appetite and proper evacuation of bowels which gradually reduces the trouble.[1]

## Leucoderma

A paste made from the seeds of the radish is valuable in leucoderma. About 35 gm. of these seeds should be powdered in vinegar and applied on the white patches of leucoderma. For better results seeds should be finely pounded along with a pinch of arsenic poison and soaked in vinegar at night. After two hours leaves will appear. It should be rubbed on the white patches of leucoderma.[2] This preparation is meant for external use only.

## Other Skin Disorders

Radish seeds contain a bleaching substance and emulsion of

1. Kvj. Ganpati Singh Verma, *Miracles of Indian Herbs,* p. 56 Rasayan Pharmacy, New Delhi; 1982.

2. Ibid., p. 92

the seeds with water applied over the face will remove black heads and freckles. It can also be applied with beneficial results in the treatment of ringworm.[3]

# Soyabean

Botanical Name : *Glycine max merr*
Indian Name : *Bhat, Soyabean*

## Description

The soyabean is one of the most nutritious foods. It belongs to the family of legumes or pulses and is perhaps one of the earliest crops cultivated by man. It is one of the most important sources of oil and protein.

The soyabean is an annual plant, upto 150 cms. in height. It has hairy, twining or climbing stems, alternate leaves and hairy, grey, brown or black, pods, borne in clusters on short stalks. Seeds are more or less round, with yellow, green, brown or black colour.

## Origin and Distribution

The name Soya has its origin in the Chinese word *shu* and *sou*. The Aryans of Central Asia considered soya along with honey as sacred food to be offered to the departed. The ancient yogis of the Indus Valley Civilisation supplemented their meatless diet with this bean to ward off deficiency of good quality protein.

The soyabean is a native of the Far East. It has been an important food crop in China. Manchuria and Korea long before the dawn of human history. It was first referred to in a Chinese book written by Emperor Shennung of China as early as 2838 BC. It was given very great importance in China so much so that the Emperor of the country to sow it every year with great pomp. It is now very popular crop of the world over and is widely cultivated in the United States, Europe, South Africa,

3. Dr. Aman, *Medicinal Secrets of Your Foods*, p. 163. *Indo American Hospital, Mysore, 1985*

Egypt, Russia, Australia and other countries. In recent years several countries like Brazil, Mexico, Rumania, Paraguay and Argentina have substantially increased their soyabean production. India too has joined the 'soyabean race' in its expansion programme and there is growing awareness among the consumers in the country of the potential uses of soyabean.

## Food Value

The soyabean is esteemed for its high food value. It is a valuable source of protein, vitamins, minerals and other food ingredients. It also contains vitamin B complex, biotin, folic acid, pantothenic acid, pyridoxine and vitamin E.

**Soyabean\***

| Food Value | | Minerals and Vitamins | |
|---|---|---|---|
| Moisture | 8.1% | Calcium | 240 mg |
| Protein | 43.2% | Phosphorus | 690 mg |
| Fat | 19.5% | Iron | 11.5 mg |
| Fibre | 3.7% | Small amounts of | |
| Minerals | 4.6% | Vitamin B Complex | |
| Carbohydrates | 20.9% | and Vitamin E | |
| | 100% | | |

\*Values per 100 gms edible portion          **Calorific Value - 432**

The soyabean is particularly valued for its high protein content of great biological value. Its protein is 'complete' as it contains all the essential amino acids or building blocks of protein in the proportions that make them most available and most valuable for human needs. It is the best of all vegetable proteins and ranks in this respect with protein of milk, eggs and meat. But soyabean contains by far more protein than these articles.

## Natural Benefit and Curative Properties

The Soyabean contains many medicinal virtues. While most of the proteins are acid in their ash, soyabean is rich in alkaline-bearing salts and hence regarded as a corrective diet. The Chinese, who consume soyabeans liberally, believe that it makes the body plump, improves the complexion, stimulates the growth and removes constipation and many other physical ailments. Modern researches carried out in the laboratories in Europe and America have corroborated much of these claims

Soyabean, especially in the form of milk, is highly beneficial in the treatment of several ailments This milk is prepared by soaking the beans in water for about 12 hours The skin of the beans is then removed and after a thorough wash, they are turned into fine paste in a grinding machine. The paste is mixed with water, three times its quantity. The milk should then be boiled on a slow fire, stirring it frequently After it becomes a little cooler, it should be strained through a piece of thin cloth and sugar be added to it.

Soyabean milk is at par in importance with cow's milk in feeding children. Investigations have shown that 90 per cent of the soyabean protein is absorbed in the body and 95 to 100 per cent of the milk is digested. Soyabean milk is very helpful in maintaining intestinal health. The soyabean curd is a health food par excellence It is better than soyabean milk in taste and aroma and it very much resembles the dairy curd The curd is prepared by allowing the milk to cool, then seeded with a small quantity of cow's milk curd or soyabean milk curd and allowed to remain for 12 hours to set. Its regular use will help maintain the intestinal health, prevent diseases arising from defective digestion and retard the ageing process.

One of the chief uses of soyabeans is as a source of lecithin, which is a great natural emulsifier. Lecithin, as is well known helps disperse deposits of fatty materials and cholesterol in certain vital organs. It is rich in substances which are important for the proper functioning of all living cells in the body. It is also an important component around brain and nerve cells. Lecithin is so abundant in soyabeans that most of the lecithin used commercially comes from them.

**Diabetes**

Soyabean contains a fairly large amount of carbohydrate but there is little or no starch in it. It is, therefore, regarded as a very suitable food for diabetic patient. Its carbohydrate produces heat and energy in the body without causing sugar to appear in the urine.

**Skin Disorders**

The soyabean is regarded as a valuable food remedy in eczema and other skin affections. It renders unnecessary the use of animal protein, that is, meat, eggs and milk and thus reduces

143

the inflammatory activities in the skin and is free from the tendency to produce sensitivity or allergic reactions which so frequently attend the users of all animal proteins. When soyabean is taken liberally, the intense itching diminishes almost immediately and disappears completely after a few days. The skin lesions also often vanish after some days. Improvement in skin health presumably occurs due to its lecithin content — a natural emulsifier which helps disperse fatty deposits and cholesterol from vital organs.[1]

### Anaemia

Soyabean, being rich in iron, has been found beneficial in the treatment of anaemia. As, however, the anaemic patients suffer from weak digestion, it should be given to them in a very light form which may be easily digested.

### Uses

Soyabeans are used in other forms such as flour, green beans, sprouts and oil. The soya flour is one of the most widely used products of soyabean. In the West, the soyabean flour industry has grown to immense proportions. The soya flour is prepared by first roasting the soyabeans and removing their coatings. They are then turned into powder. It is by far more nutritious than the wheat flour. It contains 15 times as much calcium, seven times as much phosphorus, 10 times as much iron, 10 times as much thiamine and nine times as much riboflavin as wheat flour.

### Precautions

Soyabean contains a bitter substance which can be removed by soaking soyabean in six cupfuls of warm water containing half a teaspoon of sodium bicarbonate for 10 minutes. The process also removes the colouring matter from soyabean. Soyabeans contains a factor which inhibits the action of the digestive enzyme trypsin. This factor can be destroyed by heating.[2]

1. Dr. S.J. Singh, *Food Remedies,* p. 188, Nature Cure Council of Medical Research, Lucknow, 1982.

2. Dr. Aman, *Medicinal, Secrets of Your Food,* p. 142, Indo-American Hospital, Mysore, 1985.

# Spinach

Botanical Name : *Spinacia-olerecea*
Indian Name : *Pālak*

## Description

The spinach is a leafy vegetable, with broad green leaves. It ranks high among all green vegetables. The leaves are cooling and very nutritive. This vegetable is a cool season annual crop which matures quickly. It has round, very smooth and delicate stem. The leaves are alternate, succulent, fleshy, very smooth and dark green in colour. They are generally five to eight cms. in length and one to one and half cms. in width. The bottom of the leaf is shiny, with thick veins running across.

## Origin and Distribution

The spinach is believed to have been first cultivated by the Arabs. The Persians cultivated it about 2,000 years ago. The Moors or the blacks took it to Spain from where it spread to other parts of the world. The word spinach actually comes from a Spanish word *hispania*. In India it grows in great abundance. This crop thrives best in cooler and moist climate. High humidity and cool temperature are conducive to the rapid growth of succulent, tender foliage.

## Food Value

The chemical constituents of spinach are essential amino acids, iron, vitamin A and folic acid. It is one of the cheapest vegetables which supplies the same amount of protein as one gets from the same quantity of meat, fish, eggs and chicken. Other vegetables such as tomatoes, onions and cucumbers may

### Spinach*

| Food Value | | Minerals and Vitamins | |
|---|---|---|---|
| Moisture | 92.1% | Calcium | 73 mg |
| Protein | 2.0% | Phosphorus | 21 mg |
| Fat | 0.7% | Iron | 10.9 mg |
| Minerals | 1.7% | Vitamin C | 28 mg |
| Fibre | 0.6% | Small amount of | |
| Carbohydrates | 2.9% | Vitamin B Complex | |
| | 100% | | |

*Values per 100 gms edible portion                    **Calorific Value - 17**

be added to the raw tender spinach. It will make an excellent dish with the addition of a little lemon juice and olive oil. The vitamin C content in lemon juice helps the body to absorb the entire amount of iron from the spinach consumed.

## Natural Benefits and Curative Properties

The leaves of spinach are demulcent or soothing agents, refrigerent or collants, diuretic and milk laxative.

### Constipation

Spinach juice cleans the digestive tract by removing the accumulated waste therefrom. It nourishes the intestines and tones up their movements. It is, therefore, an excellent food remedy for constipation.

### Anaemia

This vegetable is a valuable source of high grade iron. After its absorption in the system, the formation of haemoglobin and red blood cells take place. It is thus highly beneficial building up the blood and in the prevention and treatment of anaemia.

### Acidosis

Spinach is also a rich source of calcium and other alkaline elements which are essential for keeping the tissues clean and for preserving the alkalinity of the blood. It, therefore, helps prevent chronic diseases which thrive on the formation of too much acid in the system.

### Night Blindness

The spinach is particularly rich in vitamin A. It contains more vitamin A than most other green vegetables. This vitamin promotes growth and health, specially the health of the eyes. Lack of this vitamin may lead to night blindness. Spinach is thus an effective food remedy for the prevention and treatment of night blindness.

### Tooth Disorders

The spinach juice is effective in strengthening the gums and preventing and curing dental cavities. Chewing raw spinach leaves cures pyorrhoea. A mixture of carrot juice and spinach juice, taken early in the morning, can cure bleeding and ulcerated gums.

### Pregnancy and Lactation

As the richest source of folic acid, spinach is a very valuable food during pregnancy and lactation. Megaloblastic anaemia of pregnancy occurs because the mother is deficient in folic acid. This deficiency of folic acid occurs as this substance is required for the developing foetus. Regular use of spinach during pregnancy will help prevent the deficiency of folic acid. It will also prevent threatened abortion and accidental haemorrhage, deficient absorption of food by small intestine associated with lassitude i.e. tiredness, shortness of breath, loss of weight and diarrhoea. Spinach is also good source of nutrition for nursing or lactating mothers and improves the quality of their milk.

**Urinary Disorders**

Fresh spinach juice taken with tender coconut water once or twice a day acts as a very effective but safe diuretic due to the combined action of both nitrates and potassium. It can be safely given in cystitis, nephritis and scanty urination due to dehydration.

**Respiratory Disorders**

Infusion of fresh leaves of spinach prepared with two teaspoonful of fenugreek seeds mixed with a pinch of ammonium chloride and honey is an effective expectorant tonic during the treatment of bronchitis, tuberculosis, asthma and dry cough due to congestion in the throat. It sooths the bronchioles, liquifies the tenacious sputum and forms healthy tissues in the lungs and increase resistance against respiratory infections. It should be taken in doses of 30 ml. three times daily.

**Uses**

Spinach is often cooked as a green vegetable, It is also used as a soup. Small, young and tender leaves of spinach can be used as raw salads. They are as appetising as tender lettuce leaves. The leaves of spinach are so juicy that no additional water is needed for its cooking. The leaves should first be washed in several changes of water. The water which clings to the leaves is sufficient for cooking without adding more. The leaves should always be cooked on a moderate heat. It contributes roughage, colour and a bland flavour to the diet and it helps to balance the fuel foods in the menu.

It however, contains a small amount of oxalic acid which is insoluble in the fluids of the alimentary tract and is harmful in gravels, gout and liver disease. Therefore, it should not be used by those suffering from these ailments.

# Tomato

Botanical Name : *Lycopersicon-esculentum*
Indian Name : *Tamātar*

## Description

The tomato, is one of the most important vegetables in most regions of the world. It is a short-lived perennial annual plant. It has vigorous tap root, extensive fibrous roots, solid, hairy stems and spirally arranged, mainly oval leaves. The fruit is a fleshy, round or lobed, smooth or furrowed, red, pink or yellow berry with numerous flat, slightly curved seeds.

The tomato originally as a small, wrinkled thick-skinned and seedy vegetable, much smaller in size and irregular in form. Many scientific methods were employed to bring it to its present shape and quality. It has now hundreds of varieties, many of which are smoothy and globular, with almost solid pulp.

## Origin and Distribution

Tomato is considered to be a native of South America, probably the Peru-Equator. From there it was brought to Europe by the Spaniards in the early 16th century. But for several hundred years, it was grown only as a garden ornament and was called 'love apple'. Only in 1860, it was discovered that tomato was as good a food as any other fruits or vegetable. Soon after this discovery, it gradually became very popular all over the world. It is now grown in Malaysia, Indonesia, Philippines. Central, East and West Africa, tropical America, the Caribbean and throughout the tropics. It holds second place among the vegetables produced in the world, only exceeded by the potato.

## Food Value

Only about 130 years back, tomato was considered poisonous. It was regarded by many as an acid-forming food which would increase the acidity of the blood and body tissues. Because of this belief, those suffering from gout, rheumatism, arthritis and general acidosis were advised not to use it. It was also blamed to be a cancer-culprit. It was thought that it has no food value and that it supplied only colour and flavour to the diet. The latest studies in nutritional chemistry have, however, completely dispelled these baseless ideas about tomato. It is now considered to have unsurpassable nutritional and health-giving qualities. Tomato is rich in calcium, phosphorus, vitamin C and carbohydrate.

## Tomato*

| Food Value | | Minerals and Vitamins | |
|---|---|---|---|
| Moisture | 94.0% | Calcium | 48 mg |
| Protein | 0.9% | Phosphorus | 20 mg |
| Fat | 0.2% | Iron | 0.4 mg |
| Minerals | 0.5% | Vitamin C | 27 mg |
| Fibre | 0.8% | Small amount of | |
| Carbohydrates | 3.4% | Vitamin B Complex | |
| | 100% | | |

*Values per 100 gms edible portion     **Calorific Value - 20**

The carbohydrate in tomato is chiefly in the form of invert sugar which is the predigested form. It contains very small quantity of starch which is converted into sugar, chiefly dextrose during the process of ripening.

## Natural Benefits and Curative Properties

The tomato, is one of the most powerful deobstruents of the *Materia Medica*. It removes disease particles and opens natural channels of the body. It is gentle natural stimulant for kidneys and helps to wash away the toxins which cause diseases and contaminate our system. They are at their best when they are fully ripe. Their vitamin C content increase as they ripen. Tomato juice is probably one of the most widely used juices. Fresh, raw tomato juice is most beneficial and has an alkaline reaction, when digested, in concentrated form. Tomato as an external application can be used as a cosmetic. Its pulp should be applied liberally on the face and left there for an hour and then washed with warm water. Repeated daily, it will give good complexion and remove ugly-looking pimples in a short time.

### Acidosis

The tomato is essentially an alkaline vegetable. Its acid taste is due to malic acid which is about 0.5 per cent. It also contains 0.52 to 1.81 per cent citric acid and only a trace of oxalic acid. These acids in tomatoes, in combination with sodium and potassium either form sodium or potassium acid malate, citrate or oxalate. Their end products, when oxidised in the body, are carbon dioxide, water and the carbonates of potassium and sodium. The latter has alkaline reaction. Tomatoes, thus leave an alkaline ash in the process of being oxidised by the body. This increases the alkalinity of the blood and decreases the urine and neutralises the acid compounds of the body such as phosphates, urea and ammonia. It is, therefore, highly beneficial in the treatment of acidosis and other disease associated with too much acid in the system.

### Diabetes

Because of its low carbohydrate contents, it is very good food for diabetic patients and for those who want to reduce their body weight. It is said to be very effective in controlling the percentage of sugar in the urine of diabetic patients.

### Eye Disorders

Being a rich source of vitamin A, tomatoes are a dependable preventive against night blindness short sightedness and other diseases of the eye caused by the deficiency of the vitamins. Tomato leaves are useful in optic nerve and eye weakness. A small handful of the freshly plucked leaves should be covered with soft hot water for 15 minutes. The water should then strained. It forms a good tonic for the eyes and optic nerve when a teaspoonful of this water is taken before meals three times daily.

### Urinary Disorder

Eating a tomato early in the morning is found to be very effective medicine to prevent the formation of urinary calculi or stone by supplying sufficient quantity of acids and vitamins A and C. It is proved that deficiency of vitamins A and C and the recurrent urinary tract infections are among the most important factors in the formation of calculi i.e. stone. Tomato restricts the acid value of urine to 5.5 or less, thereby reducing the chances of infections by increasing the acidity of the urine.

### Obesity

Tomatoes are highly beneficial in the treatment of obesity. One or two ripe tomatoes taken early morning, without breakfast, for a couple of months is considered a safe method of reduction in weight and at the same time, it also supplies the essential food elements to preserve the health.

### Intestinal and Liver Disorders

A glassful of fresh tomato juice, mixed with a pinch of salt and pepper, taken early in the morning is considered an effective remedy for morning sickness, billiousness, sluggishness and diminished responsiveness of the liver, jaundice, indigestion, excessive formation of gas in the intestines, constipation, diarrhoea due to indigestion burning in the gastro-inestinal tract and constant burning sensation in the chest due to hiatus hernia, a condition in which stomach passes partly or completely into chest.

**Respiratory Disorders**

A glassful of fresh tomato juice mixed with honey, a pinch of powdered cardamom seeds, taken after swallowing three peeled cloves of garlic every night before going to bed, is considered highly beneficial in the treatment of tuberculosis and other lung infections. It increases the body's resistance and prevents drug resistance and the relapse which are so common in tubercular patients. In asthmatics, it reduces the congestion in the bronchioles and checks the hyper-secretion of mucous and reduces the spasms.

**Painful Joints**

The juice of the whole plant including leaves, mixed with equal quntity of *till-oil,* is heated until all the watery part is evaporated and the oil is preserved in a bottle. This oil, massaged over painful joints and sprains and fomented with dry heal gives a great relief.

# Importance of Grain Cereals

Grains are generally classified as the seeds of cereal plants. They are characterised by their smallness, hardness and low water content. Most of them belong to the family of grasses, known scientifically as the family of gramineas.

The ancient Romans called Demeter, the Greek goddes of the grains and harvests, *Ceres*. The word cereal is derived from her name. Cereals have been the staple human diet from prehistoric times because of their wide cultivation, good keeping qualities, blend flavour and great variety, Each of the cereals has characteristic properties and uses.

The cultivation of grains for human consumption was probably developed around 10,000 B.C. It signified the commencement of the era of stable civilisation from the primitive unsettled nomadic life. Ground cereal converted into bread for meal revolved soom thereafter. Cereals have been modified and improved by centuries of cultivation and selective breeding.

Cereals consist of tour essential parts, namely i) the husk, hull or chaif, the outer covering loosely attached to the grain, ii) the bran or the outer coat of the grain itself, iii) the germ or embryo and iv) the endosperm which contains nutrients comprising a considerable volume of starch, a small amount of protein and a little fat. There are numerous varieties of cereals of which the most important are rice, wheat maize, millets, oats and barley.

**Food Value**

The whole grains of all cereals have a similar chemical composition and nutritive value. They are classified as carbohydrate-rich foods, for their average carbohydrate content is 70 per cent per 100 gm. They provide energy and also some protein which is usually of good quality. The protein content of grains varies from 11.8 per cent for wheat to 8.5 per cent for rice per 100 gm. Whole cereals are good sources of calcium and iron but they are totally devoid of ascorbic acid and practically devoid of vitamin A activity. Yellow maize is the only cereal containing appreciable amounts of carotene. Whole grain cereals also contain significant amounts of B group of vitamins. For a balanced diet, cereals should be supplemented by other proteins, minerals and vitamin A and C found in nuts, seeds, milk, fruits and fresh green vegetables.

Whole grain cereals play an important role in the diet. It sprouted, they provide an increase in protein balance, as well as in all other nutrients, especially vitamin C. Their complex form of carbohydrate, when in the whole state, is valuable for digestive needs, especially in providing excellent sources of vital fibre.

## Natural Benefits and Curative Properties

All grains can be ground into flour for baking nourishing breads, cookies and cakes. In prehistoric days, flour was used when fresh food was scarce; even then it was only used immediately and being freshly ground, so that it contained most of the original nourishment of the grain. The modern-day use of steel mills has resulted in a very fine grade of flour, with the consequence considerable loss of nutrients. Thus the modern grain, loses so much nourishment when hulled, refined, ground, sterilised and bleached that the result is a grossly undernourished powder.

Wheat is by far the most popular flour, but there is significant difference between whole meal wheat and plain white wheat flour. In the refining process of whole wheat, the precious wheat germ, which is the very life of grain, is removed. The wheat germ contains the all important vitamin E. The refining of grains to retain only the endosperm has a commercial basis as the refined material appears cleaner, tastes better and is easier in making breads, pastries and other delicacies. But the refined products made after the removal of germ and bran, lack sufficient bulk and leads to numerous degenerative diseases and even cancer.

153

# Barley

Botanical Name : *Hordeum vulgars*
Indian Name : *Jau*

## Description

Barley is the fourth important cereal crop in the world and sixth in India. It is very nutritious and an excellent body-builder. Barley resembles wheat in composition although it is less palatable. The Balrely grain, also called 'pearl barley', is prepared by removal of the outer husk.

## Origin and Distribution

Barely was the first cereal to be domesticated in the Middle East at least 9,000 years and was probably the most important of the early cereals. Hulled Barley was grown by the ancient Egyptians. It is now widely grown in Europe, arid regions near the Sahara and the high plateau of Tibet. The world's largest producers are the Soviet Union, Germany, China and the United States.

## Food Value

Barley is very nutritious and a rich source of protein and B-complex vitamins. Its protein quality is superior to the protein of corn and beans.

Most of the world's barley crop is converted into malt. It is most important grain used in the brewing of beer. Barley cannot be used for leavened bread because of low gluten content. It is much used in soups. Barley is also widely used as feed for live stock.

### Barley*

| Food Value | | Minerals and Vitamins | |
|---|---|---|---|
| Moisture | 12.5% | Calcium | 26 mg |
| Protein | 11.5% | Phosphorus | 215 mg |
| Fat | 1.3% | Iron | 3 mg |
| Fibre | 1.2% | Vitamin C | 5 mg |
| Minerals | 3.9% | Small amount of | |
| Carbohydrates | 69.6% | vitamin B Complex | |
| | 100% | | |

*Values per 100 gms edible portion          **Calorific Value - 336**

## Natural Benefits and Curative Properties

Barley has many medicinal virtues. Pearled barley, which is the form the grain is largely eaten and consumed as a food by invalids. The malt prepared from barley is used in the preparation of malt extract for the incorporation in the diet of the infant and the invalid.

The partially germinated and dried grain is the source of malt extract which is more nutritious than the unmalted barley. Malt extract consists chiefly of dextrin and malt sugar and contains the ferment diastase enzyme which is developed during the malting process. This ferment diastase possesses the power of converting starch into dextrin and sugar, thus assisting in the digestive of starchy or farinaceous foods.[1]

### Digestive System Disorders

The pearl barley has always been used by orient traditional physicians for the healing and the rejuvenation of the digestive system. A simple, yet effective folk remedy was to make a barley brew and sip throughout the day, while restricting intake of other foods. This folk remedy has helped many people even to this day.

The barely brew is prepared by boiling one-quarter cup of all natural pearled barley in about 2.5 litres of water. When the water has boiled down to about 1.25 litres, it should be strained carefully. This all-natural barley brew helps digestive rejuvenation in two ways. It has a demulcent or soothing response and relieves the burning digestive actions. It has also a mucilagenous response and introduces a natural oily substance which helps to protect the abraded mucous membrane of the digestive system. Once the digestive system is thus soothed and healed, it can promote better assimilation of foods.[2]

### Fevers

Barley is also useful in fevers and all inflammatory conditions on account of its soothing properties.

### Urinary Disorders

Barley gruel with butter milk and lime juice is an excellent

---

1. Dr. S.J. Singh, *Food Remedies,* p. 43, Nature Cure Council of Medical Research, Lucknow, 1982.

2. Carlson Wade, *Health Secrets from the Orient, p. 59-60, Allied Publishers Private Ltd., Bombay.*

diuretic carbohydrate food. It is highly beneficial in the treatment of urinary disorders like nepthritis and cystitis.[3]

# *Maize*

Botanical Name : *Zea manys*
English Name : Indian corn
Indian Name : *Makka*

## Description

Maize is the most important cereal in the world after wheat and rice. It is, unique among cereals. The grains are borne in separate inflorescences, which are completely enclosed as modified leaf sheaths or husks, so that it is incapable of dispersing its sheets. The corn is at its best when it is well filled but yet soft and tender. The tender maize is chiefly liked for its high sugar content. It has more sugar than any other corn. So the maize is called sweet corn.

## Origin and Distribution

The name maize is derived from an Arawak-Carib word. 'mahiz'. The early American civilisation were based on this crop, which made settled life possible in Mexico and Central America. Within a comparatively short time of the discovery of America, maize spread widely throughout the World and became an important source of carbohydrate food for the poorer countries.

### Maize*

| Food Value | | Minerals and Vitamins | |
|---|---|---|---|
| Moisture | 14.9% | Calcium | 10 mg |
| Protein | 3.6% | Phosphorus | 348 mg |
| Fat | 1.5% | Iron | 2 mg |
| Fibre | 0.5% | Small amount of | |
| Minerals | 2.7% | vitamin B Complex | |
| Carbohydrates | 66.2% | and vitamin E | |
| | 100% | | |

*Values per 100 gms edible portion          **Calorific Value - 342**

3. Dr. Aman, *Medicinal Secrets of Your Food*, p. 527, Indo-American Hospital, Mysore, 1985

## Natural Benefits and Curative Properties

The bread made from the maize flour is nutritious and palatable. It can be digested without difficulty. Taken at intervals, this bread helps to keep the colon clean. The dextrose produced from maize is used extensively in medicine.

### Constipation

Popcorn, made by heating the small grains, is a wholesome cereal food and is easily digested. It has everything in the orginal grains of corn content. It is not fattening and practically starch-free as in the process of popping, its starch is converted into dextrine and intermediate carbohydrates, a digestive product, which is easily assimilable. It is laxative and provides bulk to faeces. It also promotes peristalsis i.e. wave like movement by its tendency to absorb moisture. It is therefore, valuable food in constipation.

### Uses

Maize is prepared and consumed in various ways. It is usually ground and pounded. The meal may be boiled, baked or fried. The whole grain may be boiled or roasted and it may be fermented. Maize meal can be cooked with water to provide a thick mush or dough. It may be cooked with water to provide gruel, porridge or soup. Cornbread is made by mixing the meal with wheat flour. Immature cobs preferably sweet corn, are boiled and eaten as corn on the cob or the grain may be removed and eaten as a vegetable, or it may be canned. More mature cobs are roasted.

# *Rice*

Botanical Name : *Orya Sativa*
Indian Name : *Chawal*

### Description

. Rice is much-revered oriental food and the most important tropical cereal. It is the staple food of about half the human race and is often the main source of calories and the principal food of many millions of people.

Rice from which only husk has been removed, but layers of bran and most of the germ retained, is known as brown rice. Rice from which husk, germ and bran layers have almost completely been removed by power machinery is known as milled rice. Rice milled to a high degree is known as white rice. Rice from which husk, germ and bran layers have been partly removed without the use of power machinery is known as hand-pounded rice. Rice milled to a high degree and then coated with some foreign substance such as glucose or talcum is called polished rice. Paddy specially processed by steaming or soaking in water, then heated and dried, is called parboiled paddy. It can then be milled to various degrees or home pounded. It is called parboiled milled or parboiled home pounded.

## Origin and Distribution

Rice has been cultivated in south eastern Asia since ancient times where it is one of the oldest of food crops. The date or place of its domestication are not known with certainty. One of the earliest mention of rice dates back to 2800 BC, when a Chinese emperor established a ceremonial ordinance for the planting of rice that would later be used by the royal physicians for healing purposes. It was grown in ancient India as far back as in 3000 BC, when it appeared as a plant called 'Newaree'. The general consensus of opinion is that rice was domesticated in India or Indo-china and probably in southern India. Enormous quantities of rice are now grown over 90 per cent of the total area of 100 million hectares in southern and eastern Asia.

## Food Value

Starch constitutes the bulk of the rice grain. The protein content of the rice is lower than that of wheat, but is of superior

### Raw Handpounded Rice*

| Food Value | | Minerals and Vitamins | |
|---|---|---|---|
| Moisture | 13.3% | Calcium | 10 mg |
| Protein | 7.5% | Phosphorus | 190 mg |
| Fat | 1.0% | Iron | 3.2 mg |
| Minerals | 0.9% | Small amount of | |
| Fibre | 0.6% | Vitamin B Complex | |
| Carbohydrates | 76.7% | | |
| | 100% | | |

**Calorific Value - 346**

## Raw Milled Rice *

| Food Value | | Minerals and Vitamins | |
|---|---|---|---|
| Moisture | 13.7% | Calcium | 10 mg |
| Protein | 6.8% | Phosphorus | 160 mg |
| Fat | 0.5% | Iron | 3.1 mg |
| Minerals | 0.6% | Small amount of | |
| Fibre | 0.2% | Vitamin B Complex | |
| Carbohydrates | 78.2% | | |
| | 100% | | |

*Value per 100 gms edible portion      **Calorific Value - 345**

quality and utilised better by the body than the wheat protein.

The ancient and modern Oriental healers through traditional medicines have always advocated the use of natural brown rice as a key to youhful health-building. The processing removes many of the valuable B-complex vitamins and some of the minerals.

## Natural Benefits and Curative Properties

Rice has always been considered a magical healer in the East. It was originally believed to have medicinal values that could restore tranquility and peace to those who were easily upset. It has been mentioned in early Oriental writings that natural whole grain brown rice is a perfect healing food. In the ancient literature of Thailand, Burma, Malaya and Indo-China rice is mentioned as a source of health. It was also revered as a food of divine health and used in religious offerings.

Modern researches have confirmed the beliefs of ancient oriental folk physicians that the eating of brown rice is a source of serenity and tranquility. It has been shown to contain all the elements needed for the maintenance of good health.

Rice is about 98 per cent digestible. It is one of the most easily and quickly digested of all foods — being fully digested·in an hour. Rice starch is different from other grain starches as it contains 100 per cent amylopectin which is most completely and rapidly digested grain starch. This makes rice in ideal health food for those who seek speedy and healthy assimilation.

## Internal Rejuvenation

Rice protein, which comprises upto eight per cent of the grain, has a special benefit as it has eight of the essential amino acids in a delicately balanced proportions. A complete internal

159

rejuvenation takes place when rice protein is metabolised into health-building amino acids. These amino acids build resilient muscles which comes back to its original form after stretching and bending, healthy skin and hair and clearer eyesight and nourish the heart and lungs, tendons and ligaments, brain, nervous system and glandular network.

The B-complex vitamins, especially thiamin, riboflavin and niacin offered by natural brown rice promote youthful energy and nourishment to skin and blood vessels. An abundance of minerals in natural brown rice help to nourish the hormonal system, heal wounds and regulate blood pressure. Rice also offers iron to enrich the bloodstream and phosphorus and potassium to maintain internal water balance along with other nutrients. Rice thus helps restore internal harmony.

### High Blood Pressure

Rice has a low-fat, low-cholesterol and low-salt contents. It makes a perfect diet for those hypertensive persons who have been advised salt-restricted diets. It has been noted by modern researchers that wherever rice is used as the main food, there is a corresponding benefit of youthful vitality and a very low rate of hypertension. Calcium in brown rice, in particular, soothes and relaxes the nervous system and helps relieve the symptoms of high blood pressure.

### Body Balance

The rice diet, in combination with milk, creates a marvellous body balance. In this regimen, natural brown rice is used as the only solid food throughout the day. Fresh milk is taken with each of the rice meals. The rice may be cooked in any manner but no salt should be used. The milk should be comfortably cool. The nutrients in the rice form a unique balance with those in the milk. The two notable amino acids, isoleucine and lysine in the milk are greatly strengthened by rice protein, thereby enabling them to form stronger body-building blocks. The natural lactic acid in milk works with rice protein to aid in the absorption of iron.

### Digestive System Disorders

Rice has a very low fibre content, and is therefore extremely soothing to the digestive system. This makes rice an ideal food for digestive system disorders. Thick gruel of rice mixed with a glassful of butter-milk and a well-ripe banana given twice a day is a very nutritious diet in typhoid, gastric ulcer, gastritis, stomach and intestinal cancer, colitis, diarrhoea, dysentery, piles, rectal fissure, indigestion, in acute febrile diseases related to fever, hepatitis or inflammation of liver, jaundice, morning sickness, acute dilatation of the stomach, burning and indigestion due to hiatus hernia, excessive accumulation of the gas in the intestines, and all the diseases where the mild and light diet is indicated.

### Diarrhoea in Children

Rice is useful in treating diarrhoea in children. A teaspoonful of powder of charred par-boiled rice mixed with a glassful of butter-milk should be given in doses of an ounce every half an hour in this condition. This will bring excellent results.

### Skin Inflammation

Rice may also be used externally in the form of powder or poultice. The rice flour, dusted thickly over the surface, has a very cooling and soothing effect in small-pox, measles, prickly heat and other inflammatory affections of the skin including burns and scalds. It allays heat and irritation. Rice powder should be used soon after the occurrence of injury in case of burns and scalds and it should be dusted thickly over the whole of the affected surface.

### Uses

Rice is usually cooked by boiling in water, or by steaming, and is eaten mostly with pulses, vegetables, fish or meat. There are two varieties of rice, the long grain rice and the short and medium grain rice. When cooked, the grains of long variety soften but do not stick to each other. This variety is especially good for consuming it with curries, stews or as a side dish with a sauce or gravy Short and medium varieties have short, plump grains which cook tender and moist, with the particles tending to cling together. They are especially good for making puddings.

# Wheat

Botanical Name : *Triticum sativum*
Indian Name : *Gehun*

## Description

Wheat is one of the most common cereals used throughout the world. It is also one of the most valuable cereals and a good source of energy. With its essential coating of bran, vitamins and minerals, it is an excellent health-building food.

## Origin and Distribution

Wild species of wheat have been reported from the archaeological site of Tell Mureybat on the banks of the Euphrates, dated at about 800 BC. and at Ali Kosh in south-western Iran in deposits dated between 7500 and 6750 BC and at Hacilar in West central Anatolia at about 7000 BC. Although the earliest cultivation was apparently confined to the Near East, the wheat soon became widespread. From its early cultivation in the Balkans, wheat spread to other parts of Europe. Species of wheat appeared in India, probably before the fourth millenium BC, and in China sometime before the beginning of the Christian era. Wheat has been cultivated in India for over 5,000 years. India now ranks fourth among the topmost wheat producing countries. High yielding varieties of wheat have been developed through research.

## Food Value

Wheat has become the principal cereal, being more widely used for the making of bread than any other cereal because of the quality and quantity of its characteristic protein, called gluten.

### Whole Wheat Flour*

| Food Value | | Minerals and Vitamins | |
|---|---|---|---|
| Moisture | 12.2% | Calcium | 48 mg |
| Protein | 12.1% | Phosphorus | 355 mg |
| Fat | 1.7% | Iron | 11.5 mg |
| Minerals | 2.7% | Small amount of | |
| Fibre | 1.9% | Vitamin B Complex | |
| Carbohydrates | 69.4% | | |
| | 100% | | |

**Calorific Value** - 341

## Refined Wheat Flour*

| Food Value | | Minerals and Vitamins | |
|---|---|---|---|
| Moisture | 13.3% | Calcium | 23 mg |
| Protein | 11.0% | Phosphorus | 12.1 mg |
| Fat | 0.9% | Iron | 2.5 mg |
| Minerals | 0.6% | Small amount of | |
| Fibre | 0.3% | Vitamin B Complex | |
| Carbohydrates | 73.9% | | |
| | 100% | | |

*Value per 100 gms edible portion          **Calorific Value - 348**

As it is gluten that makes bread dough stick together and gives it the ability to retain gas, the higher the proportion of gluten in the flour, the better for making leavened bread.

The germ or embryo of the wheat is relatively rich in protein, fat and several of the B vitamins. So is the scutellum in wheat, which contains 50 times more thiamin than the whole grain. The outer layers of the endosperm and the aleurone contain a higher concentration of protein, vitamins and phytic acid than the inner endosperm. The inner endosperm contain most of the starch and protein in the grain.

Wheat is usually ground into flour before use as food. In ancient times, wheat grains were crushed between two large stones. This method of stone-grinding preserved all parts of the kernel and the product was called 'whole wheat'. If it is finely ground, it becomes whole wheat flour. The value of stone grinding is that the grain is ground slowly and it remains unheated, and a whole food. In modern times steel roller mills have superseded stone grinding. These mills grind wheat hundred times faster, but they impoverish the flour by removing the wheat germ, resulting in colossal loss in vitamins and minerals in the refining process.

## Natural Benefits and Curative Properties

The wheat, as produced by nature, contains several medicinal virtues. Every part of the whole wheat grain supplies elements needed by the human body. Starch and gluten in wheat provide heat and energy; the inner bran coats, phosphates and other mineral salts; the outer bran, the much-needed roughage— the indigestable portion which helps easy movement of bowels; the germ, vitamins B and E; and protein of wheat helps build and repair muscular tissue. The wheat germ, which is removed in the process of refining, is also rich in essential vitamin E, the lack of which can lead to heart disease. The loss of vitamins and minerals in the refined wheat flour has led to widespread prevalence of constipation and other digestive disturbances and nutritional disorders. The whole wheat, which includes bran and wheat germ, therefore, provides protection against diseases such as constipation, ischaemic, heart disease, disease of the colon called diverticulum, appendicitis, obesity and diabetes.

Dr. Ann Wigmore, founder director of the Hippocrates Health Institute, Boston, U.S.A. is one of the proponents of the 'wheat grass therapy'. According to her, "guided by spiritual mentality and nourished only by live uncooked food, the body will run indefinitely, unhampered by sickness". Dr. Wigmore utilises the chlorophyll present in wheat grass as a body cleanser, rebuilder and neutraliser of toxins.[1] Wheat grass juice furnishes the body with vital nourishment, providing extra energy to the body. This juice contains nearly 70 per cent of chlorophyll. It is also a rich source of vitamin A, B and C. It also contains minerals like calcium, iron, magnesium, phosphorus, potassium, sodium, sulphur, cobalt and zinc.

Chlorophyll, one of the main constituents of wheat grass is very beneficial for the body. Chlorophyll, due to its high vitamins and mineral contents, purifies blood. This property is used by the body to cleanse and rebuild itself. By drinking this juice regularly, toxins can be neutralised. It thus helps to maintain good health.

**Tooth Disorders**

Wheat is valuable in the prevention and cure of pyorrhoea. It takes time to eat wheat and as it is generally taken with other foods, it compels the chewing of other foods also. This not only provides the needed exercise for the teeth and gum but also a great aid to digestion.

Wheat grass juice acts as an excellent mouth wash for sore throats and pyorrhoea. It also prevents tooth decay and tooth aches. Therefore it is beneficial to chew wheat grass which draws out toxins from the gums and thus checks bacterial growth.

---

1. Dr. Ann Wigmore, *Be your Own Doctor*, p. 5, Hemisphere Press inc, New York.

## Constipation

The bran of wheat, which is generally discarded in milling of the flour, is more wholesome and nourishing than the flour itself. It is an excellent laxative. The laxative effects of bran are much superior to those of fruits or green vegetables as cellulose of the latter is more easily broken down by bacteria while passing through the intestine.[2] The bran is highly beneficial in the prevention and treatment of constipation due to its concentration of cellulose which forms a bulk-mass in the intestines and helps easy evacuation due to increased peristalsis.

## Skin Diseases

It has been scientifically proved that chlorophyll arrests growth and development of harmful bacteria. Wheat grass therapy can be effectively used for skin diseases and ulcerated wounds as by retarding bacterial action, it promotes cell activity and normal re-growth. By drinking wheat grass juice regularly, an unfavourable environment is created for bacterial growth. Poultice of wheat grass juice can be applied on the infected area, as it is an able sterilizer.

Externally, wheat flour is useful as a dusting powder over inflamed surface as in burns, scalds and various itching and buring eruptions. Whole wheat flour, mixed with vinegar, boiled and applied outwardly removes freckles.[3]

## Digestive System Disorders

Wheat grass juice used as an enema helps detoxify the walls of the colon. The general procedure is to give an enema with lukewarm or neem water. After waiting for 20 minutes, 90 to 120 ml. of wheat grass juice enema is given. This should be retained for 15 minutes. This enema is very helpful in disorders of the colon, mucous and ulcerative colitis, chronic constipation and bleeding piles.[4]

## Circulatory Disorders

The chlorophyll content present in wheat grass enhances heart and lung functions. Capillary activity also increases while toxaemia or blood poisoning is reduced. Due to increased Iron

2. Dr. S.J. Singh, *Food Remedies*, p. 211, Nature Cure Council of Medical Research, Lucknow, 1982.

3. Ibid, p. 209

4. Dr. T. Chandrashekar, *Wheat Grass Juice,* article in Health Herald, Bangalore, January, 1986, p. 11.

content in the blood and haemoglobin, lungs function better, Oxygenation improves and the effect of Carbon-dioxide is minimised. It is for this reason that wheat grass juice is prescribed for circulatory disorders.

Wheat grass is grown by soaking a good variety of wheat for eight to 10 hours. The water should then, be draind and grains be allowed to sprout for 15 hours. Earthen pots or wooden trays can be used to grow the wheat grass. These trays should be filled with compost manure. The wheat sprouts should be spread and the trays should be covered with a dark cloth or the trays kept away from the sunlight in a room. These trays should be sprinkled with water once or twice a day and they should be allowed to stay as such for six to seven days until the grass grows five to seven inches high.

Chewing wheat grass is the easiest method to drink wheat grass juice. As an alternative to chewing, wheat grass should be cut finely and ground in a grinder with addition of water to enable the extraction of the wheat grass juice. This juice should be drunk within 10 to 15 minutes after extraction. In the early stages of wheat grass therapy about 100 ml. to 150 ml. of wheat grass juice should be taken daily. As the body becomes accustomed to its taste, the quantity of wheat grass juice can be gradually increased until the intake is about 250 ml. to 300 ml. per day. Wheat grass juice should be mixed thoroughly with saliva before being swallowed slowly. This juice should be drunk an hour before a meal and two to three hours after the meal.

**Uses**

*Chappatis* are the common form in which wheat is eaten in India, Pakistan and Iran. They are made from whole wheat flour, called *atta*. Wheat taken in the shredded form called *dalia* is extremely wholesome. It has been a very favourite Indian dish in olden days. It is cooked by soaking two tablespoonful of crushed or shredded wheat for half an hour and then cooking it on slow fire till the water nearly dries up. Thereafter milk and honey may be added to taste. It is a nourishing morning breakfast food item.

# Importance of Pulses

Pulses may be defined as the dried edible seeds of cultivated legumes. They belong to the family of peas, beans and lentils. The English word pulse is taken from the Latin *puls,* meaning pottage or thick pap. The pulses are a large family and various species are capable or surviving in very different climates and soils.

Traces of pulse crops have been found from ancient times in archaeological sites of both the Old and New Worlds and they appear to have been among the earliest domesticated plants. These findings indicate an almost simultaneous arrival of cereals and pulses around 10,000 BC.

Pulses are cultivated in all parts of the world, and they occupy an important place in human diet. They however, make a much more important contribution to the diet of all classes of society in the East than in the West. In India especially, people who are mostly vegetarian depend largely on cereals and pulses as their staple food, which serve as the main source of dietary protein and energy.

### Food Value

Pulses contain more protein than any other plant. They serve as a low-cost protein to meet the needs of the large section of the people. They have, therefore, been justifiably described as 'the poor man's meat'. Their low moisture content and hard testa or seed-coat permit storage over long periods. In addition to providing dry pulses, many of the crops are grown for their green edible pods and unripe seeds. Nutritionally, immature fruits have distinctly different properties to those of the mature seed; the protein content is lower but they are relatively richer in vitamins and soluble carbohydrates. The leaves and shoots of some of the crops are used as pot-herbs.

In general, pulses contain 20 to 28 per cent protein per 100 gm. with the exception of soyabean which has as much as 47 per cent. Their carbohydrate content is about 60 per cent per 100 gm. except soyabean which has about 30 per cent. Pulses are also fairly good sources of thiamin and niacin and provide calcium, phosphorus and iron. On an average 100 gram of pulses contain energy 345 kcal, protein 24.5 gm., calcium 140 mg., phosphorus 300 mg., iron 8 mg., thiamin 0.5 mg., riboflavin 0.3 mg. and niacin 2 mg.

## Natural Benefits and Curative Properties

The nutritive properties of pulses resemble in many respects those of the whole cereal grains; but there are important differences. First, the pulse protein is low in sulphur containing amino acids, but rich in lysine in which many cereals are deficient. A combination of pulses and cereal proteins may, therefore, have a nutritive value as good as animal proteins. Secondly, pulses as a class are good sources of the B group of vitamins except riboflavin. More important, the greater part of these vitamins present in the harvested seeds is actually consumed. There are no losses comparable with those that may arise in the milling and cooking of cereals. Pulses are therefore, an excellent preventive against beriberi.

Thirdly, although pulses, like cereal grains, are devoid of vitamin C, large amount of ascorbic acid are formed on germination. Sprouted pulses are, therefore, an important food which will protect against scurvy. Dietitians in Asian and African hospitals make beneficial use of sprouted pulses for their menus, especially when fresh vegetables and fruits are scarce or too expensive.

In health, the digestion of pulses and the absorption of their principal nutrients is practically complete and nearly as effective as is the assimilation of cereals. Their digestion, may, however, be incomplete in gastro-intestinal disorders. Only small qantities of well-cooked pulses should, therefore, be included in the diets of patients with stomach disorders.

## Uses

Pulses are used as a common foodstuff in various forms. Pulses, dehusked, decorticated and whole seed, are used as *dhal* and taken with *chappatis* and cooked rice, Whole seeds take longer time to cook than the dehusked and decorticated ones which are relatively better digestible.

Pulses are also commonly used in the form of flour such as that of Bengal gram, green gram, black gram, known as 'besan'. It is used for mixing with cereal flour in various proportions for *chappatis* and other preparations.

The practice of utilizing germinated seed or sprouting or young seedlings of pulses as a fresh vegetable is widespread in the Orient. The storage of dried seed and their sprouting as required enables a continuous supply of fresh vegetable material to be produced. There is an amazing increase in nutrients in sprouted pulses when compared to their dried embryo. In the process of sprouting, the vitamins, minerals and protein increase substantially with corresponding decrease in calories and carbohydrate content.

Sprouting of the pulses not only improves nutritive value but also digestibility. During sprouting, starch is broken down to dextrin and maltose, and proteins are broken down to polypeptides, peptides and amino acids. Some of the bound iron is converted to a more readily assimilable form. Phosphorus is liberated from phytate. The ascorbic acid or vitamin C content rises from negligible levels in the seed to 12 mgs. per 100 grams after 48 hours of germination. Riboflavin and niacin contents increase significantly. These changes are brought about by enzymes which become active during germination.

## *Bengal Gram*

Botanical Name : *Cicer arietinum*
Other English Name : *Chick-pea*
Indian Name : *Channā*

### Description

Bengal gram is one of the most important pulses in India. It is consumed in the form of whole dried seeds and in the form of dhal, prepared by splitting the seeds in a mill and separating the husk. Seeds are angular with pointed beak and small hilum. All parts of the plant are covered with glandular hairs.

## Origin and Distribution

Bengal gram is believed to have originated in western Asia. It spread at a very early date to India and Europe. The crop was known to the ancient Egyptians, Hebrews and Greeks. Its areas of cultivation are India, Burma, Pakistan, Egypt and other Mediterranean countries, Ethiopia, South America and tropical Australia.

## Food Value

The whole dried Bengal gram seeds are cooked or boiled. They are also consumed raw after soaking them in water. For preparation of *dhal*, the seeds are sprinkled with water and heaped overnight to soften the husk and are then dried before milling. Flour is made by grinding seeds. This flour is one of the main ingredients of many forms of Indian confectionary made with *ghee* and sugar. It is also used for preparing many tasty snacks like *sev, chila* and *pakoras* and curries like *koftas*. Green pods and tender shoots are used as a vegetable.

### Bengal Gram (Whole Dried Seeds)*

| Food Value | | Minerals and Vitamins | |
|---|---|---|---|
| Moisture | 9.8% | Calcium | 202 mg |
| Protein | 17.1% | Phosphorus | 312 mg |
| Fat | 5.3% | Iron | 10.2 mg |
| Minerals | 3.0% | Vitamin C | 3 mg |
| Fibre | 3.9% | Small amount of | |
| Carbohydrates | 60.9% | Vitamin B Complex | |
| | 100% | | |

Calorific Value - 360

### Bengal Gram (dhal made from Seeds)*

| Food Value | | Minerals and Vitamins | |
|---|---|---|---|
| Moisture | 9.9% | Calcium | 56 mg |
| Protein | 20.8% | Phosphorus | 331 mg |
| Fat | 5.6% | Iron | 9.1 mg |
| Minerals | 2.7% | Vitamin C | 1 mg |
| Fibre | 1.2% | Small amount of | |
| Carbohydrates | 59.8% | Vitamin B Complex | |
| | 100% | | |

*Value per 100 gms edible portion          Calorific Value - 372

## Natural Benefits and Curative Properties

Bengal gram has many medicinal properties. Soaked i water overnight and chewed in the morning with honey, th whole gram seed acts as a general tonic. The liquid, obtained b soaking the seeds and then macerating them, also serves as tonic. Sprouted Bengal gram supply plenty of B-complex and vitamins. Cooked germinated gram is a wholesome food f children and invalids. However, excessive use of Bengal grar causes indigestion and may precipitate urinary calcium due t high concentration of oxalic acid and form urinary stone calculi.

### Diabetes

Experiments have shown that the intake of water extract Bengal gram enhances the utilization of glucose in both—th diabetic and the normal persons. Tests were conducted CFTRI Laboratories in Mysore, on a chronic diabetic patien whose insulin requirement was of the order of 40 units a day When kept on a diet which included liberal supplements o Bengal gram extract, the condition of the patient improved considerably and his insulin requirement was reduced to abou 20 units per day. Diabetic patients who are on a prescribed die which does not severely restrict the intake of carbohydrates, but includes liberal amounts of Bengal gram extract, have shown considerable improvement in their fasting blood sugar levels, glucose tolerance, urinary excretion of sugar and general condition.

### Anaemia

Fresh juice of Bengal gram leaves is a very rich source of iron. It is, therefore, highly beneficial in the treatment of iron-deficiency anaemias. A tablespoonful of fresh juice mixed with honey should be taken in this condition.

### Digestive System Disorder

An acid liquid is obtained by collecting the dew drops from the leaves by spreading a thin white cloth over the crop at night or by any other means. This acid liquid contains about 94 per cent malic acid and 6 per cent oxalic acid and is used medicinally. It is a valuable astringent for use in dyspepsia, vomiting, indigestion, costiveness, diarrhoea and dysentery.

## Painful Menstruation

A bath prepared by putting the entire Bengal gram plant in hot water is highly beneficial in painful menstruation. It may be taken in the form of a sitting steam bath.

## Skin and Hair Disease

Flour of the unroasted Bengal gram is a very effective cleansing agent and its regular use as a cosmetic bleaches the skin. In allergic skin diseases like eczema, contact dermatitis, scabies, washing the skin with this flour will be highly beneficial. The Bengal gram flour can be beneficially used in the treatment of pimples. The flour should be mixed with curd to make a paste. This paste should be applied to the face. It should be washed off after some time. Washing the hair with Bengal gram flour, keeps them clean, soft and free from hair diseases.

## Sexual Dysfunction

Flour of the puffed Bengal gram is a very nutritive food, and an effective remedy for impotency and premature ejaculation. For better results, two tablespoonful of this flour should be mixed with sugar, powdered dates and skimmed milk powder. It can be packed in airtight tins and used when required.

# Black Gram

Botanical Name : *Phasleolus mungo*
Indian Name : *Urad*

## Description

Black gram is one of the most highly prized pulses of India. It is an erect, sub-erect or trailing, densely hairy annual herb. The tap root produces a branched root system with smooth, rounded nodules. The pods are narrow, cylindrical and upto 6 cms. long. It is the most nutritious of all pulses.

## Origin and Distribution

Black gram originated in India where it has been in cultivation from very ancient times. It is not known in a wild state. It has been introduced in recent times elsewhere in the tropics, mainly by Indian immigrants. It occurs throughout

Asia and in Africa and the western India, but nowhere it is so important as in India.

**Food Value**

Black gram is boiled and eaten whole or after splitting into *dhal*. It is extensively used in various culinary preparation like idli, curries and papad. The green pods are eaten as vegetables and they are highly nutritious. The hulls or the outer covering of gram and straw are used as cattle feed.

Black Gram*

| Food Value | | Minerals and Vitamins | |
|---|---|---|---|
| Moisture | 10.9% | Calcium | 154 mg |
| Protein | 24.0% | Phosphorus | 385 mg |
| Fat | 1.4% | Iron | 9.1 mg |
| Minerals | 3.2% | Small amount of | |
| Fibre | 0.9% | Vitamin B Complex | |
| Carbohydrates | 59.6% | | |
| | 100% | | |

*Value per 100 gms edible portion          **Calorific Value - 347**

## Natural Benefits and Curative Properties

Black gram is demulcent or soothing and cooling agents. It is an aphrodisiac and nervine tonic. However, excessive use of black gram causes flatulence which can, however, be prevented by adding little asafoetida, pepper and ginger in the culinary preparations. It should not be taken by those who are easily predisposed to rheumatic diseases and urinary calculi as it contains oxalic acid in high concentration.

### Diabetes

Germinated black gram, taken with half a cupful of fresh bitter gourd juice and a teaspoonful of honey is highly beneficial in the treatment of milder type of diabetes. It should be used once daily for three to four months with restriction of carbohydrates Even in severe cases, regular use of this combination, with other precautions, is useful as a health giving food for the prevention of various complications that may arise due to malnutrition in diabetic patients.

### Sexual Dysfunction

Black gram *dhal* soaked in water for about six hours and then fried in pure cow's ghee, after draining the water is an excellent sex tonic. It can be used with wheat bread and honey with highly beneficial results in functional impotency, premature ejaculation and thinness of the semen.

### Nervous Disorders

The above preparation eaten with half boiled egg is an excellent tonic in nervous disorders such as nervous weakness, weakness of memory, schizophrenia and hysteria.

### Hair Disorders

Washing the hair with a paste of cooked black gram dhal and fenugreek lengthens the hair, keeps them black and cures dandruff.

### Digestive System Disorders

Black gram is valuable in digestive system disorders. In the form of decoction, it is useful in dyspepsia, gastric catarrh, dysentery and diarrhoea.

### Rheumatic Afflictions

A liniment made from black gram is useful as an external application in rheumatism, contracted knee and stiff shoulder. It is prepared by boiling about 4 Kgs. of black gram pulse in 38.4 litres of water. It should be boiled down to about 9.6 litres and strained. The strained decoction should be boiled with about 2.5 litres of sesame oil and 1/2 kg. of rock salt till the water has been evaporated. Paste of the fresh root is also useful in rheumatic pains.

## *Green Gram*

Botanical Name : *Phaseolus aureus*
Indian Name : *Mung*

### Description

The green gram is one of the most wholesome among pulses in India. It is free from the heaviness and tendency to flatulence, which is associated with other pulses.

### Origin and Distribution

This plant is a native of India and since ancient times it has been in cultivation. It is not found in a wild state. It was introduced early into Southern China, Indo-China and Java. It has been introduced in comparatively recent times into East and Central Africa, the West Indies and the United States.

**Food Value**

The green gram forms a very nutritious article of diet. It is consumed in the form of whole dried seeds and in the form of *dal*, prepared by splitting the seeds in a mill. The sprouted *mung* beans are a highly nutritious food. The beans are soaked overnight, drained and placed in containers in a dark room. They are sprinkled with water every few hours and the sprouts are ready in about three days. One pound of dry beans gives six to eight pounds of sprouts. There is an amazing increase in nutrients in sprouted beans when compared to their dried embryo.

### Green Gram (Whole dried Seeds)*

| Food Value | | Minerals and Vitamins | |
|---|---|---|---|
| Moisture | 10.4% | Calcium | 124 mg |
| Protein | 24.0% | Phosphorus | 326 mg |
| Fat | 1.3% | Iron | 7.3 mg |
| Minerals | 3.5% | Small amount of | |
| Fibre | 4.1% | Vitamin B Complex | |
| Carbohydrates | 56.7% | | |
| | 100% | | |
| | | **Calorific Value - 334** | |

### Green Gram (Dal)*

| Food Value | | Minerals and Vitamins | |
|---|---|---|---|
| Moisture | 10.1% | Calcium | 75 mg |
| Protein | 24.5% | Phosphorus | 405 mg |
| Fat | 1.2% | Iron | 8.5 mg |
| Minerals | 3.5% | Small amount of | |
| Fibre | 0.8% | Vitamin B Complex | |
| Carbohydrates | 59.9% | | |
| | 100% | | |

*Value per 100 gms edible portion    **Calorific Value - 348**

## Natural Benefits and Curative Properties

Cooked *dal* of green gram is a very digestive food for invalid and sick persons. Its regular use during childhood, pregnancy and lactation helps one to get the required nutrition and promote health. It is an aperient i.e. a laxative, when given in large quantities. The soup made from it is the best article of diet after recovery from acute illness.

Applied in the form of powder, it is said to be useful in relieving the heat or burning of the eyes. A poultice of this powder is useful for checking secretion of milk and reducing distention of the mammary glands.

### Fevers

Water in which green grams are soaked is an excellent medicine during cholera, measles, chicken-pox, small-pox, typhoid and all types of fevers. It can be given in a small quantity even during acute phase of appendicitis.

### Beauty-Aid

Flour of the green gram is an excellent detergent and can be used as a substitute for soap. It removes the dirt and does not cause any skin irritation. Its application over the face bleaches the colour and gives good complexion. Black gram flour is also used for washing the hair with green gram paste to lengthen hair and prevent dandruff.

### Uses

The dried beans are boiled and are eaten whole or after splitting into *dhal*. They are parched and ground into flour after removal of the testa or the seed-coat. This flour is used in various Indian and Chinese dishes. The green pods are eaten as a vegetable. In China and the United States it is used for bean sprouts.

# *Pigeon Pea*

Botanical Name : *Cajanus cajan*
Other English Name : *Red gram*
Indian Name : *Arhar*

### Description

The pigeon pea is one of the important pulses in India. It is a woody, short-lived perennial shrub, 1 to 4 metres tall. It is sometimes grown as an annual herb It has a pronounced deep

176

tap-root, angled and hairy stems, and spirally arranged leaves. The fruit is a flattened pod. Seeds vary in size, shape and colour, usually round or oval, white or greyish, red, brown purplish or speckled, with a small white hillium.

**Origin and Distribution**

Pigeon pea is probably a native of tropical Africa, where it is sometimes found wild or naturalized. Seeds have been found in Egyptian tombs and it was cultivated there before 2000 BC. Pigeon peas were cultivated in Madagascar from very early times, and this region now constitutes a centre of diversity with the greatest number of varieties. The crop was taken to the New World in early post-columbian days, but it did not reach the Pacific until 1772. Pigeon peas are now widely spread throughout the tropics and subtropics. Its areas of cultivation include India, Malaysia, Indonesia, Philippens, The Carribean, East and West Africa.

**Food Value**

The fresh leaves are used, as a vegetable. The immature pods are also cooked. Dried seeds are added to soups and stews. The ripe dry seeds are boiled and eaten as a pulse. In India these are split into *dhal*. The dried husks, seeds and broken *dhal* are used as cattle feed in India.

**Pigeon Pea***

| Food Value | | Minerals and Vitamins | |
|---|---|---|---|
| Moisture | 13.4% | Calcium | 73 mg |
| Protein | 22.3% | Phosphorus | 304 mg |
| Fat | 1.7% | Iron | 5.8 mg |
| Minerals | 3.5% | Small amounts of | |
| Fibre | 1.5% | Vitamin B Complex | |
| Carbohydrates | 57.6% | | |
| | 100% | | |
| *Value per 100 gms edible portion | | **Calorific Value - 335** | |

## Natural Benefits and Curative Properties

The pigeon pea is easily digested and therefore suitable for invalids. It has many medicinal properties. It relieves inflammation of internal organs. However, excessive use of pigeon pea causes hyper-acidity and wind in the intestines. Therefore, it is forbidden in gastric ulcer and heart disease.

### Baldness

A fine paste made of this pulse is highly useful in bald patches. It should be applied regularly.

### Jaundice

The expressed juice of the leaves given, with a little salt, is highly beneficial in the treatment of jaundice. 60ml of this juice should be taken daily in this condition.

### Checking Breast Milk Secretion

The pulse and leaves ground into a paste, warmed and applied over the mamma, has the effect of checking the secretion of breast milk.

### Inflammation

The leaves of the plant are effective in all inflammatory conditions. A poultice made with the seeds will also reduce swelling.

### Piles

Paste of the leaves, mixed with a teaspoonful of paste of neem leaves, is highly beneficial in the treatment of piles and itching in the anus. It should be taken once daily for a week.

# Importance of Nuts and Seeds

Nuts and seeds are the most important and potent of all foods. Nuts are also seeds from which trees grow if they remain in the ground until they germinate. Seeds have always been considered as the symbol of resurrection. It contains the embryo, the reproductive power which is of vital importance for the lives of human beings and their health. Dead, dry, hard and tough—it appears quite lifeless. But given moisture and soil, it will sprout again and will produce not one but many more seeds or nuts.

Nuts include a number of fruits, containing one or more kernels within a hard shell of woody fibre. There are a variety of nuts. The most popular among them are almond, cashewnut, coconut, groundnut, pistachio and walnut. All the available varieties contain a concentrated food of high nutritional value.

### Food Value

Seeds contain all the important nutrients needed for human growth. They are excellent sources of protein and the essential unsaturated fatty acids which are necessary for health. They are also one of the best natural sources of lecithin, most of the B-complex vitamins and vitamin E, which are perhaps the most important elements for the preservation of health and prevention of premature ageing. Besides, they are rich sources of minerals and supply the necessary bulk in the diet.

Similarly, genuine nuts are high in protein, fat and carbohydrate foods. They are rich in many minerals such as potassium, the healer, sodium, the preserver of youth, calcium and phosphorus which are essential for strong bones and teeth and sulphur which purifies and activates the body. Raw nuts are generously supplied with B vitamins, which are valuable for the brain and nervous system as well as vitamin F needed for alround development. Some of them also contain vitamin A and C. The general composition is roughly formed by protein 10 to 25 per cent, fat 40 to 60 per cent, carbohydrate 10 to 20 per cent, cellulose three to five per cent and minerals nearly two per cent per 100 grams.

## Natural Benefits and Curative Properties

Seeds contain pacifarins, an antibiotic resistance factor, which increases man's natural resistance to disease. They also contain auxones, natural substances which help produce vitamins in the body and play an important role in the rejuvenation of cells, thereby preventing premature ageing.

Sprouted seeds are excellent live nourishment. They are valuable sources of protein, vitamins, and complex carbohydrates. Germinated seeds enormously increase their nutritional value. All seeds should ideally be eaten raw but those, which can be sprouted, should be consumed in that form to derive maximum nutrition.

However, nuts should be used in their natural raw state. Raw nuts are among the foods highest in fat. But the fat of nuts is completely natural and unprocessed which is best for the body. It is especially rich in linoleic acid and is least damaging to heart and arteries.

Nuts often produce oil half their weight. The high energy value of the nuts is mainly due to their oil content. They render approximately 600 calories per 100 grams compared to 348 for wheat, 346 for lentils, and 283 for dates of equal weight. The nut oil is used for cooking all over the world. Pure nut oils are often used in medicine.

Raw nuts are safe food as their hard shell offers an effective barrier against bacteria. They can be preserved with all their nutritional value intact for long periods in their natural unshelled state. Being extremely low in water content, nuts have excellent storage qualities. They can be kept fresh for many years in sealed containers provided they are held in a cool dry place.

An excellent way of using nuts is to take it in the form of butter. The nut butter is easily digested. It can be prepared at home by removing the skin of the nuts and then grinding them into fine paste. It should, however, be ensured that unheated and unsalted nut butters are used. They can be put on fruits for added protein, in dressings and added to soups at the end of cooking or used in vegetables. Nut butters are especially beneficial for older persons who do not like meat and cannot eat it because of lack of teeth or dentures that are painful. Their **B** vitamins, minerals and proteins act in the digestive tract and improve the appetite.

The most easily digested form of nut is, however, nut milk drinks. They make rich non-acid-forming drinks, full of nourishment. Blanched nuts may be soaked in water for few hours. This softens the structure of the nut kernel. Then 90 gm. of soaked nuts may be put in 150 ml. of water and kept for two or three minutes in a liquifier. They may be flavoured with honey or any kind of fruit concentrate. The fluid resembles dairy milk in composition and appearance. It is so easily digested that it may be used in baby feeding with advantage. Almond milk especially makes a very alkaline drink, high in protein and easy to assimilate and absorb.

The nut milk can be used in various ways. It can be used as *sherbet* by adding sugar and lime juice. The milk may be curdled like the dairy milk with the addition of a little curd.

# *Almond*

Botanical Name : *Prunus amygdalus*
Indian Name : *Badam*

**Description**

The almond, known as the king of nuts, is a highly nutritious food. It is rich in almost all the elements needed by the body. It is an effective health-building food, both for the body and mind, and a valuable food remedy for several common ailments.

There are two varieties of almonds, the sweet and the bitter. There are thin-skinned and thick-skinned among the sweet variety. The thin-skinned, known as *Kagzi* in vernacular, is the best for use. The bitter variety of almonds should not be used as they contain prussic acid, a deadly poison. They have, however, some commercial importance and are used for producing almond oil, perfume and cosmetics.

## Origin and Distribution

Almond is a native of Morocco. It has been cultivated from ancient times. The Romans called it the 'Greek nut'. It was grown in Syria and Palestine during the days of the Bible. It is now grown in several parts of the subtropical regions, especially in Morocco, Italy, France, Portugal, California and Australia. It is also cultivated in Southern Africa and many parts of Asia.

Its cultivation in India is mostly confined to Kashmir and some areas of Himachal Pradesh which border Tibet.

## Food Value

Almonds are one of the best nut and seed foods. The best way of using almonds is to soak them in water and grind them into fine paste of the blanched almonds i.e., after peeling of the skin. This paste is called almond butter. It is easily assimilated and is preferred to dairy butter by many vegetarians. This butter is of special value to older people who are generally bothered with the problem of not getting enough protein in their diets. By taking almond butter, they will be able to get not only high quality protein but also other excellent food ingredients, contained in the almond, in the most easily digestible form.

### Almonds*

| Food Value | | Minerals and Vitamins | |
|---|---|---|---|
| Moisture | 5.2% | Calcium | 230 mg |
| Protein | 20.8% | Phosphorus | 490 mg |
| Fat | 58.9% | Iron | 4.5 mg |
| Minerals | 2.9% | Niacin | 4.4 mg |
| Fibre | 1.7% | Small amount of | |
| Carbohydrates | 10.5% | Vitamin B Complex | |
| | 100% | | |
| *Value per 100 gms edible portion | | Calorific Value - 665 | |

The most useful preparation of almonds is the almond milk. It can be easily prepared by grinding the blanched almonds —i.e. almonds without outer coat to a smooth paste and adding cold boiled water to the consistency of the milk. With the addition of little sugar, it makes a delicious and nutritious drink. One kilogram of milk may be obtained from 250 grams of almonds. The almond milk can be converted into curd and butter as in case of ordinary milk.

The almond milk is rich in vitamins. It possesses certain

advantages over the ordinary milk. It is more easily digestible than the cow's milk and is useful for the children with whom the cow's milk does not agree.

The fat in almonds is unsaturated and as such they provide one of the most beneficial kinds of fat. In specific terms, every 100 grams of almonds contain 11 grams of linolenic acid. This fatty acid is one of the most polyunsaturated and highly beneficial in lowering serum cholesterol levels.

## Natural Benefits and Curative Properties

The medicinal virtues of almonds arise chiefly from pharmaco dynamic action of copper, iron, phosphorus and vitamin $B_1$. These chemicals exert a synergic action — i.e. increased energy due to chemical interaction and help the formation of new blood cells, haemoglobin and play a major role in maintaining the smooth physiological functions of brain, nerves, bones, heart and liver. The almond is thus highly beneficial in preserving the vitality of the brain, in strengthening the muscles and in prolonging life. It forms a vital part of all tonic preparation in Ayurveda and Unani Medicines.

Paste of almonds with milk cream and fresh rose bud's paste applied daily over the face is a very effective beauty aid. It softens and bleaches the skin and nourishes it with the choicest skin-food. Its regular application prevents early appearance of wrinkles, black heads, dryness of the skin, pimples and keeps the face fresh.

A teaspoonful of almond oil mixed with a teaspoonful of *amla* juice, massaged over scalp, is a valuable remedy for falling hair, thinness of hair, dandruff and premature graying of hair. Almonds should be consumed properly for beneficial results. The skin of almonds should always be removed before use as it contains irritating properties. This can be done by soaking them in water for one or two hours.

Almonds should be thoroughly chewed and they should not be eaten immediately after meals. They are a very concentrated food, with high calorific value. They should, therefore, be mostly used with bulky vegetables and fruits like raw turnips, lettuce, cucumbers and apple.

## Anaemia

Almonds contain copper in organic form at the rate of

1.15 mg. per 100 grams. The copper along with iron and vitamins, acts as a catalyst · in the synthesis of blood haemoglobin. Almonds are, therefore, a useful food remedy for anaemia.

## Constipation

The use of almonds has proved highly beneficial in the treatment of chronic constipation. It is an excellent laxative. 11 to 15 kernels taken at bed time will facilitate a clear motion the next morning. Those who suffer from weak stomach can take seven grams of almond oil with hot milk.

## Impotency

Almonds are very useful in case of loss of sexual energy which usually results from nervous debility and brain weakness. Their regular use will strengthen sexual power. Chewing of equal quantity of almond kernels and roasted gram also help in restoring sexual vigour.

## Skin Disorders

Wild almonds are considered useful in skin diseases, especially eczema. For this purpose, a few leaves of the wild almond are pulverised with water and the cream so prepared is applied to the affected parts. Almonds are also beneficial in the treatment of pimples. In this conditon, the endocarp which is hard cover of the seed, should be ground with water and applied over the affected parts. In case of inflammatory condition of the skin, the external application of almond oil will ease the pain and cool the heat.

## Respiratory Diseases

An emulsion of almonds is useful in bronchial diseases, hoarseness and tickling cough. It is prepared by pounding the nuts and mixing the powdered kernels with orange or lemon juice. A teaspoonful of the oil given with 10 drops each of fresh white onion juice and ginger juice, daily thrice for a fortnight, is useful in whooping cough, bronchitis and asthma.

# Coconut

Botanical Name : *Cocos nucifera*
Indian Name : *Narial*

## Description

The coconut is known as a 'wonder-food'. It is a near perfect diet, as it contains almost all the essential nutrients needed by the human body. It is also considered a sacred fruit and holds a very high place in all religious ceremonies.

The coconut is 20 to 30 cm. long, somewhat three-sided. The outermost part of the fruit is green and shining when tender. It becomes rough and matty after its maturity. It is almost entirely water-proof and very hard. Beneath this is a thick layer of stout fibres, the layer being at times over 25 mm. in thickness. Then follows a hard, stonelike layer, about 6 mm. thick. The inside of this stony layer is lined with a fairly thick coating of soft, milky-white flesh. The cavity inside the flesh is filled with a watery fluid. It grows on a tall stately, unbranched tree, with a terminal crown of leaves, growing to a height of 20 to 30 m.

## Origin and Distribution

Coconut is believed to have originated in the Indo-Malaya region and to the south west of New Guinea. It was taken to the mainland of Asia in prehistoric times. There is evidence that the coconut was grown in India about 3,000 years ago. The *Vedas* describe coconut tree as *Kalpa-Vriksha* or the tree of heaven. According to Hindu mythology when Lord Vishnu, the God protector of universe, came to this earth, he brought with him the *Karpagavalli* or the coconut tree which means giver of all health, energy, strength, tranquillity, longevity and peace. Coconut is held in very high esteem in all religious ceremonies. It is offered as a token of devotion while celebrating *pooja* in temples of various deities.

Coconut reached East Africa, and possibly Panama before 1492. Thereafter, it gradually spread to all the tropical areas of the world. It is now widely cultivated in India, Sri Lanka, Indonesia, Philippines, the East Indies, the West Indies, and the islands of the Indian and Pacific Oceans. Coconut tree grows abundantly along the entire coast of the sea and it thrives well in loose sandy soil. Its age varies from 80 to 200 years.

## Food Value

The coconut is highly nourishing, strengthening and fattening food article. The coconut has a high oil content which is easily digestible. It is more easily utilised by the body than all other fats. This oil closely resembles the butter in physical and chemical properties. The protein content of coconut is of high quality, containing all the amino-acids. It is also rich in potassium, sodium, magnesium and sulphur. The energy value of the dried coconut is very high, being 662 calories per 100 grams.

### Coconut*

| Food Value | | Minerals and Vitamins | |
|---|---|---|---|
| Moisture | 36.3% | Calcium | 10 mg |
| Protein | 4.5% | Phosphorus | 240 mg |
| Fat | 41.6% | Iron | 1.7 mg |
| Minerals | 1.0% | Vitamin C | 1 mg |
| Fibre | 3.6% | Small amount of | |
| Carbohydrates | 13.0% | Vitamin B Complex | |
| | 100% | | |

**Fresh Coconut's Calorific Value - 444**
**Dried Coconut's Calorific Value - 662**

*Values per 100 gms edible portion

## Natural Benefits and Curative Properties

The coconut is nourishing, strengthening and fattening dietary. It is used in all stages of maturity. As a food, it is most valuable before it matures. Its jelly-like tender kernel contains various enzymes and is easily digestible. Ripe kernel is rich in fat and carbohydrates. It does not have high protein like other nuts and can be taken with vegetable salads and cooked green vegetables. It is, however, difficult to digest with starches. The milk of fresh coconut forms a valuable food for children suffering from nutritional deficiency. It has a greater vitamin A content than the coconut itself. It has adequate natural minerals and a high quality protein which are valuable for growth and repair of the body.

The water of the tender green coconut, generally known as mineral water, is used as a beverage and a refreshing drink. A tender coconut, which is fully grown and only one month old, contains about 400 to 465 C.C. of water. It contains sufficient sugar in an easily assimilable form. It is an excellent tonic for health. The water of a single coconut contains sufficient vitamin C to meet the daily requirements of the body. It also contains several vitamins in the B group. These are niacin, pantothenic acid, biotin, riboflavin, folic acid and thiamin as well as pyridoxin in traces. The water also contains sodium, potassium, calcium, magnesium, iron, copper, phosphorus, sulphur and chlorine.

### Intestinal Worms

The coconut is an ancient and very effective remedy for intestinal worms of all kinds. A tablespoonful of the freshly ground coconut should be taken at breakfast, followed by a dose of castor oil after three hours. The process may be repeated till the cure is complete.[1]

### Acidity

The mature dried coconut is valuable in the treatment of acidity. Its oil reduces the acid secretion of the stomach and gives much relief to the patient.

### Digestive System Disorder

Tender kernel of coconut is highly beneficial in the treatment of digestive system disorders. It is valuable in diseases like indigestion, colitis, gastric ulcers, diarrhoea, dysentery and piles. The tender coconut water is also an excellent remedy for flatulence, vomiting and dyspepsia. In vomiting, it is food medicine of great value when other methods of allaying it have failed.

### Dry Cough

Coconut milk, mixed with a tablespoonful of poppy seeds, milk and pure honey one tablespoonful, taken every night before going to bed, is an effective food remedy for dry cough due to throat irritation or due to excessive smoking.[2]

### Cholera

Tender coconut water is very useful in cholera. Eight to 12 ounces of this water mixed with a teaspoonful of fresh lime juice

---

1. Dr. S.J. Singh, *Food Remedies*, p. 74, Nature Cure Council of Medical Research, Lucknow, 1982.

2. Dr. Aman, *Medicinal Secrets of Your Food,* p. 482, Indo-American Hospital, Mysore, 1985.

should be administered orally to the patient. It rectifies the electrolyte balance and neutralises the acidosis of the blood. Coconut water is a known source of potassium-rich fluid, and since cholera patients can almost invariably take oral fluids following initial correction of shock and acidosis, the experts suggest intake of coconut water is a must for cholera patients.[3]

## Urinary Disorders

The coconut water is valuable in urinary disorders. It acts as a natural diuretic in heart, liver and kidney disorders such as scanty and suppressed urination, albuminuria that in presence of protein in urine, dropsy and high acidity of urine.

## Bilious Fever

Coconut water is highly beneficial in the treatment of bilious fever. It should be given frequently in small doses. Water should, however, not be taken immediately after taking coconut water. It may be taken after some time, if necessary.

## Ascites

It is a disease which causes swelling in the stomach due to fluid accumulation. Coconut water is valuable in ascites. The patient should be given two or three glassful of coconut water to drink. This quantity may be increased or decreased according to the condition and the needs of the patient.

## Skin Disorders

The oil extracted from the flesh of the ripe nut is an effective dressing for burns and scalds. It is of great value in the preparation of ointments as it penetrates the skin readily. The tar-like fluid obtained from the red, hot shell of a ripe nut is a rubifacient which causes reddening and warming of the skin. It is a household remedy for ringworm, itch and other skin diseases.[4]

## Uses

The coconut is widely used in the preparation of many products. The oil is the most important of these products. It is used in cooking and made into coco jam, coco butter, margarine, vegetable butter and salad oil. The oil is a hair-restorer and is

3. Ibid., p. 485.

4. J.F. Dastur, *Medicinal Plants of India and Pakistan*, p. 61, D.B. Taraporevala Sons & Co. (P) Ltd., Bombay, 1985.

used as a hair oil in all parts of the country. Dried coconut is used in cooking and in various preparations of sweets and curries. The milk from a dried coconut is a fine medium of cooking in place of ghee or oil.

# Groundnut

Botanical Name : *Arachis hypogaea*
Other English Names : *Peanut, Monkeynut, ground pea*
Indian Name : *Mongphali*

## Description

The groundnut belongs to the pea and bean family and is a legume. But it is considered as nut because of its high nutritional value. That is how it is used in family meals and snacks.

The groundnut is the only nut that grows below the earth. The groundnut plant is a variable annual herb, which grows upto 50 cm. in height. The flowers of the plant develop a stalk which enters into the soil, forms a pod containing generally two seeds. They become mature in about two months, when the leaves of the plant turn yellow. The plant is then removed from the earth and allowed to dry. After three to six weeks they are separated from the plant.

## Origin and Distribution

The groundnut is a native of South America, where it has been cultivated for several centuries. It has been found in the excavations dated 1,000 BC in coastal Peru. In the 16th century, the Portuguese took it from Brazil to West Africa and Spaniards took it across the Pacific to the Philippines. From there, it spread to China, Japan, Malaysia and India and as far as Madagascar. India leads the world in groundnut production and about 40 per cent of the groundnut entering the world commerce is from India.

## Food Value

The groundnut is particularly valued for its protein contents, which is of high biological value. Kg. for Kg., groundnuts contain more protein than meat—about two and a

189

half times more than eggs, and far more than any other vegetable food except soyabean and yeast. The proteins in groundnut are well balanced, except for slight deficiency in some of the essential amino acids. As it happens, these amino acids are abundant in milk which can be combined with groundnut products for better results.

For proper digestion, groundnut requires thorough mastication. Experiments made with the groundnut show that it is quite indigestible unless chewed to a smooth paste. This difficulty is obviated by roasting them. The baked raw starch increases its digestibility. As an alternative to chewing it can be ground into a paste which on account of its richness in fat, is called 'peanut butter'. A little salt is generally added to it. A little peanut oil is also put if it becomes dense.

### Groundnut*

| Food Value | | Minerals and Vitamins | |
|---|---|---|---|
| Moisture | 3.0% | Calcium | 90 mg |
| Protein | 25.3% | Phosphorus | 350 mg |
| Fat | 40.1% | Iron | 2.8 mg |
| Minerals | 2.4% | Vitamin E | 261.4 mg |
| Fibre | 3.1% | Small amount of | |
| Carbohydrates | 26.1% | Vitamin B Complex | |
| | 100% | | |
| Values per 100 gms edible portion | | Calorific Value - 567 | |

## Natural Benefits and Curative Properties

Groundnut is one of the most nourishing foods available in the world. The U.S. Department of Agriculture considers it having maximum five important nutrients such as food energy, protein, phosphorus, thiamin and niacin.

Hence apart from their nutritional value, groundnuts have considerable medicinal value. They contain a good deal of oil which is very easily digested and for this reason they are useful consumptives. The oil is regarded as an excellent aperient or a mild laxative and emollient which softens the skin. Eating fresh roasted groundnuts with jaggery and goat's milk is a very nutritious food for growing children, pregnant women and nursing mothers. It builds a resistance against all infections, particularly tuberculosis and hepatitis.

However, excessive use of groundnuts causes high acidity in the body, spermetorrhoea and premature ejaculation. Some persons are allergic to roasted groundnuts. Asthmatics in particular should abstain from eating groundnuts in excess. Groundnuts that are boiled in salted water are less harmful for such persons. Liberal use of groundnuts should also be avoided by persons with gastritis and jaundice as their excessive use causes hyperacidity of the stomach, indigestion and heart burn.

## Excessive Bleeding

Several groups of researchers in England have reported using groundnuts or groundnut products in the treatment of haemophilia, an inherited blood disease which causes haemorrhage. Beneficial results have also been reported from the use of groundnuts in severe cases of epistaxis or nose bleeding and in cases of excessive bleeding during menstruation in women.

## Obesity

Groundnuts are considered beneficial in the treatment of obesity. Experiments have shown that weight can be reduced by eating a handful of roasted groundnuts with tea or coffee without sugar an hour before lunch time. It reduces appetite and thus reduces the weight gradually.

## Diabetes

Groundnuts are valuable in diabetes. Eating a handful of groundnuts daily by diabetics will not only prevent malnutrition, particularly the deficiency of niacin, but also checks the development of vascular complications.

## Diarrhoea

Groundnuts are also useful in diarrhoea, especially chronic diarrhoea which is more frequent immediately after meals. The patients can benefit greatly by drinking goat's milk in which lemon is squeezed with a handful of fresh roasted groundnuts. This type of diarrhoea is caused due to nicotinic acid deficiency. The groundnuts, which has required quantity of niacin, are valuable in this disease.

## Teeth Disorders

Chewing fresh groundnuts with a pinch of salt strengthens the gum, cures stomatitis, kills harmful bacteria and safeguards the enamel of the teeth. The mouth should, however, be washed with water after eating groundnuts.

**Beauty Aid**

Groundnut oil can serve as a beauty aid. A teaspoon of refined groundnut oil, mixed with equal quantity of lime juice, may be applied daily on the face once before going to bed. It keeps the face fresh. Its regular use nourishes the skin and prevents acne.

**Uses**

The groundnuts are consumed in many ways and various forms. They may be eaten raw, boiled, steamed or roasted. They are sometimes eaten as a sweetmeat by coating them with sugar. In the West, they form an important constituent of confections. They are often taken in the form of nut chocolates, candies and sandwiches.

A large number of food products are prepared from the groundnuts. The groundnut flour is becoming increasingly popular in the West. It is by far superior to wheat flour in nutritive value. Groundnuts may be used for preparing a nutritive and tasty milk. About one pound of lightly roasted nuts may be soaked in water for about two hours. The skin of the nuts should be removed by rubbing in water. The soaked nuts are made into a fine paste in a stone grinder. The paste is mixed with water to the quantity of three times the bulk of the paste. It should be strained through a thin cloth before use. The milk may be boiled without loss of its food value. Sugar may be added to taste. In food value and composition, the peanut milk is similar to dairy milk and may be used as its substitute.

The groundnut milk may be converted into curd. A small quantity of the cow-milk curd may be added to the milk and allowed to remain overnight to set. It tastes like milk curd and possesses much of its qualities.

Groundnuts are often used as vegetables when the seeds are still tender. They may also be taken in their germinated form. Germination not only renders them more digestible, but also enhances their food value, especially in their vitamin B and C contents.

# Mustard Seeds

Botanical Name : *Brarrica nigra*
Indian Name : *Raye*

## Description

The mustard is a well-known oil seed. It is a small annual plant which grows upto a height of one metre with some branches. It has round stem with long intermodes, simple, alternate and very soft yellowish green leaves. The fruit is a pod of about 2.5 cms. long containing seeds.

Dry mustard seeds are small, measuring about 1 mm. in diameter. They are round and darkish-brown or greyish-brown in colour. They have no smell, but when pounded and moistured with water, they emit a peculiar pungent odour. The taste of the mustard seeds is bitter and pungent.

## Origin and Distribution

Black mustard is a native of Eurasia. It has been in cultivation in Europe for a long time. This was the first species to provide table mustard for use as a condiment. It has been used by Romans, Greeks and Indians since ancient times. The plant is cultivated as a field crop in most temperate countries.

## Food Value

The mustard seeds are used as condiment throughout India. The seeds yield 28 per cent of a fixed oil which is used in medicine and soap-making. The seeds also contain about one per cent of a volatile oil which is used as a counter-irritant when greatly diluted. The oil extracted from the seeds is used in North India as a hair oil, for frying and other cooking purposes. It is also used in pickles and salads. In Punjab, Delhi and Western Uttar Pradesh, the leaves are used as a vegetable.

## Natural Benefits and Curative Properties

Mustard seeds as well as its oil is used in many prescription for the treatment of various ailments. White mustard seeds can be used beneficially as a beauty aid. A handful of these seeds are roasted in a litre of sesame or coconut oil. The oil is then strained and cooled. It is applied with little water over face before going to bed. It will cure pimples and whiten the complexion.

Mustard oil boiled with henna leaves is useful in healthy

growth of hair. About 25 grams of mustard oil should be boiled in a tinned basin. A little quantity of henna leaves should be gradually put in this oil till about 60 grams of these leaves are thus burnt in the oil. The oil should then be filtered through a cloth and stored well in a bottle. Regular massage of the head with this oil will produce abundant hair.

### Poisoning

Mustard seeds have emetic properties which cause vomiting. A teaspoonful of seeds, mixed in a glassful of water, generally produces free vomiting in five to 10 minutes. This is especially useful in drunkenness, narcotic and other poisonings.

### Muscular Pains

Mustard is a rubefacient which causes reddening and warming of the skin. Its plaster or paste made with water, is applied as analgesic in rheumatism, sciatica, paralysis of limbs and other muscular pains. The plaster should, however, never be directly applied to the skin as it may cause painful blistering. A layer of lint material should be put between the mustard paste and the skin.

### Convulsion in Children

A teaspoonful of powdered mustard seeds mixed in a gallon of warm water is used as therapeutic bath in convulsion of children caused by high fever.

### Ringworm

Mustard paste as an external application is highly beneficial in the treatment of ringworm. This paste should be applied after washing the skin with sufficiently hot water.

## Safflower Seeds

Botanical Name : *Carthamus tinctorius*
Indian Names : *Kusum, Kusumbha, Karadai*

### Description

The safflower is an important oil-seed crop. It is a highly-branched, glabrous, annual plant, 0.5 to 1.5 m. tall. It has long and stout taper root and spirally arranged, dark green and glossy leaves. Florets are tubular and usually orange-yellow in colour. Safflower seeds are bitter in taste and look more or less like the seeds of orange.

## Origin and Distribution

Safflower is believed to have originated in an area bounded by the eastern Mediterranean and the Persian gulf. It has been identified as growing in Egypt 4,000 years ago. Safflower has been cultivated in Egypt, the Middle East and India initially for the orange dye obtained from the florets. It is still used as dye in India. It spread throughout the Mediterranean region and eastwards to China and Japan. Safflower was taken early by the Spaniards to Mexico. It was introduced experimentally as an oil crop in the United States in 1925, where it has been grown on a commercial scale since 1950, particularly in California. In Sanskrit literature of ancient India, safflower has been described as *kusumbha*, from which the most common modern name of *kusum* is derived. Kusumbha oil was regarded as purgative and identical properties were assigned to it in Egypt, Africa and India. It is now cultivated for oil in parts of North Africa, India, China, the United States and Australia.

## Food Value

The oil content of the seeds varies from 20 to 38 per cent. The thinner the hull the greater will be the oil content. The drying oil has a high linoleic acid content, about 75 per cent, and a very low linolenic acid content. The crude protein content of the expressed meal or cake varies from 20 to 55 per cent, depending on the amount of hull removed during processing.

## Natural Benefits and Curative Properties

Safflower oil is one of the most polyunsaturated. The medicinal value of linoleic acid came into prominence in the latter 1960s following the publication of the findings of researchers in a series of medical and scientific journals. These findings proved that this fatty acid was highly beneficial in lowering serum cholesterol levels in laboratory animals and humans. From virtual obscurity safflower oil became a best-seller within a few years. This is no wonder, with its very high linoleic acid content.

It has also been discovered that linoleic acid promotes and improves availability of calcium to the body's cells, thereby virtually acting as a vitamin. Some scientists refer to it as "vitamin F".

## Heart Disease

Safflower oil has proved beneficial in lowering blood cholesterol. Hence it can be used liberally by persons suffering from cardio vascular disorders. An emulsion by trade name Saffloxin-cipla is used routinely during myocardial infraction, cardiac ischaemia and hypertension.

## Constipation

One teaspoonful of kernel of the seeds, taken with six shelled almonds and honey has proved highly beneficial in the treatment of constipation. It has been found to be a safe laxative for the young, weak and pregnant women. A very popular Unani laxative medicine called *Twarishe Qhurtum* is prepared from safflower seeds.

## Sexual Debility

Safflower seeds are highly beneficial in the treatment of sexual debility. For better results, powder of the dry seeds should be mixed with pistachio nuts, honey and almonds. It should be used with milk once before going to bed. It is a very effective aphrodisiac. It improves sexual vigour and thickens semen.[1]

## Asthma

Safflower seeds are highly beneficial in the treatment bronchial asthma. Half a teaspoon of powder of the dry seeds, mixed in a tablespoonful of honey, can be taken once or twice with great benefit in this disease. It acts as an expectorant and reduces the spasms by liquefying the tenacious sputum. Infusion of the flowers mixed with honey is also useful in asthma.[2]

## Female Disorders

A decoction prepared by boiling two teaspoonfuls of powdered seeds in 120 ml. of water is given as a remedy to cure painful menstruation. Dried flowers mixed with rose are also given as a medicine in this condition. A brew made from safflower foliage is said to prevent abortion and the female sterility.

1. Hakeem Mohammad Musa, *Random Notes,* p. 180, Urdu MS. *Kachiguda,* Hyderabad, 1901.

2. Dr. Aman, *Medicinal Secrets of Your Food,* p. 520, Indo-American Hospital, Mysore, 1985.

## Eczema

It has been established in laboratory animal tests that eczem can result from lack of linoleic acid. Safflower oil can thus b beneficially used in the treatment of this disease. Tw tablespoonful of safflower oil should be taken daily in thi condition. The quantity can be reduced to one tablespoonfu after the condition improves.

# *Sesame Seeds*

Botanical Name : *Sesamum indicum*
Other English Name : *Gingelly Seeds*
Indian Name : *Til*

## Description

The sesame is a well known oilseed. It is probably the oldest of all cultivated seed crops. It has been regarded as a food of high value throughout Asia since ancient times.

Sesame is a variable annual herb, one to two metre tall, covered with glandular hairs and with a somewhat foetid or pungent smell. The seeds are small, smooth, white, red or black.

## Origin and Distribution

Sesame originated in Africa. It has been identified in the excavation at Harappa, Pakistan, dating to 2000 BC and was recorded in Egypt about 1300 BC at the time of the expulsion of the Israelites. Its seeds and oil have been widely mentioned in Indian literature from the Vedic period and was used for religious ceremonies such as *shraddha* and *pitryana.* It spread early through West Asia to India, China and Japan. It is now widely grown in parts of Latin America also.

## Food Value

Sesame seed kernels are a nourishing food. The hard husk of sesame seeds must be removed prior to consumption, for it is abrasive on the intestines and rather bitter, due to its high concentration of oxalic acid. The husk is also very rich in calcium, iron and vitamin B1, but these are unfortunately non-extractable by human digestive means.

## Natural Benefits and Curative Properties

There are three varieties of sesame seeds; black, white and red. The balck variety yields the best quality of oil and is also best suited for medicinal purposes. The white seeds are extremely rich in calcium and are useful in all cases of calcium deficiency. The red variety is exceptionally rich in iron. The seeds are emollient that softens the skin, nourishing tonic, emmenagogue that stimulates menstruation, demulcent or soothing, laxative, diuretic and fattening.

The oil extracted from sesame seeds is of very high medicinal quality. Charak, the great medical authority of ancient India, has said that of all the oils, the gingelly or sesame oil is the best. It has the finest flavour and a high boiling point. This latter quality is important from the health point of view, for it indicates that less molecular restructuring takes place in sesame oil than any other seed oil.

### Piles

Sesame seeds are highly beneficial in the treatment of piles. They can be taken in the form of decoction or as sweet-meats. Ground to paste with water, they are given with butter for bleeding piles.

### Skin Disorders

A poultice of the seasame seeds can be applied externally with beneficial results over ulcers, burns and scalds. External application of a mixture of equal parts of sesame oil and lime water is also effective in these conditions. The oil is also used as a substitute for olive oil in pharmaceutical preparations for external uses.

### Anaemia

Black sesame seeds, as a rich source of iron, are valuable in anaemia. An emulsion of the seeds is prepared by grinding and straining them after soaking them in warm water for a couple of hours. This emulsion, mixed with a cupful of milk and sweetened with jaggery, should be given to patients suffering from anaemia.

### Dysentery and Diarrhoea

Sesame seeds are useful in dysentery and diarrhoea. Two tablespoonfuls of the seeds should be lightly roasted on a frying pan. They should then be ground into fine powder and mixed with one tablespoon of cow's ghee. The mass should be divided into three parts. Each part should be used with boiled goat's milk thrice daily for six days by the patients suffering from chronic dysentery or diarrhoea. It acts as an excellent medicine in these conditions.

### Abortion

Sesame seeds are traditionally used as a medicine for causing abortion. One tablespoonful of the seeds should be ground with equal quantity of palm jaggery and used twice daily in the early stage of pregnancy for this purpose. It excites the uterine contractions and thus expels the fertilized ovum.

### Respiratory Disorders

The seeds are valuable in respiratory disorders. An infusion of sesame seeds, mixed with a tablespoonful of linseed, a pinch of common salt and a desertspoonful of honey, should be given once at night with beneficial results, in acute and chronic bronchitis, pneumonia and asthma. It acts as an expectorant.

### Menstrual Disorders

Half a teaspoon of powder of sesame seeds taken with hot water twice daily acts excellently in reducing spasmodic pain during menstruation in young unmarried anaemic girls. Its regular use, two days prior to the expected periods, cures scanty menstruation. Warm hip bath containing a handful of bruised sesame seeds should be simultaneously taken along with this recipe.

### Hair Disorders

Crushed leaves of sesame are considered beneficial in the treatment of dandruff. A decoction made from the leaves and root is used as a hair wash. It is said to prevent premature greying of hair and promote their growth.

### Uses

Sesame is grown for its edible seeds which are the source of gingelly oil. This oil is used as a substitute for olive oil as a salad dressing and in cooking. The fried seeds are eaten in soups and, mixed with sugar, are a popular sweetmeat in Africa and Asia.

# Sunflower Seeds

Botanical Name : *Helianthus annus*
Indian Name : *Suryamukhi*

## Description

Sunflower seeds are probably the most familiar of all edible seeds. They are the tightly packed core of the glorious sunflowers. The flowers have gigantic size, yellow in colour and they always keep their face towards sun. The seeds are commonly crushed for their oil. There are many varieties of sunflower seeds. The larger kernels are generally used for edible purposes while the smaller for crushing into edible oil.

## Origin and Distribution

The sunflower is believed to have originated in Mexico area. Sunflower was introduced in Europe in the 16th century. It became very popular as an ornamental flower and was established as an oilseed crop in Eastern Europe. It was imported into Russia from Holland in the 18th century. The first commercial production of oil began in 1830-40. The crop steadily grew in importance and soon became one of the world's most important oilseeds.

## Food Value

Sunflower kernels are well above average in protein, phosphorus and iron concentration. They are very rich sources of B-complex vitamins.

Sunflower seeds can be used to enrich any meal. They can be sprinkled over cereals, salads, yogurt and soups. They can be mixed with vegetables to augment their protein, vitamin and mineral contents. They can be used like chopped nuts on desserts. They can also be taken as snacks between meals.

## Natural Benefits and Curative Properties

Sunflower seed kernels are an excellent protein food and can be considered as complete food. Eaten with milk, the seeds contribute to the needs of protein, the substance of which every cell of the body is made. The kernels contain almost 50 per cent fat which makes them a highly satisfying food that prevents the let-down feeling of fatigue and weariness which are due eating too much carbohydrate and sugar.

200

Being rich in potassium, the seeds help balance the sodium in our diets, thereby protecting the body from the dangers of too much salt in tissues. Magnesium being plentiful in sunflower, it helps the heart and other muscles as well as nervous tissues in the maintenance of proper balance between magnesium and calcium.

## High Cholesterol level

The seeds contain substantial quantity of linoleic acid which is the fat helpful in reducing cholesterol desposits on the walls of arteries. Substituting sunflower seeds for some of the solid fats like butter and cream will, therefore, lead to great improvement in health.

## Beriberi and Pallagra

As a rich source of thiamin and niacine, sunflower seeds help to protect the health of nerves and brain as well as skin and digestive tract. Lack of these vitamins will produce deficiency like beriberi and pallagra.

## Anaemia

The flour made from sunflower seeds is one of the richest sources of iron in any food. It is, therefore, highly beneficial in the prevention and treatment of anaemia.

## Respiratory Diseases

Powder of the dry seeds or the decoction of the pounded seeds is used as a remedy for bronchitis, laryngitis, tonsillitis, influenza and cough. It is believed that growing sunflower in the home garden prevents influenza and cold.

# Curd

Other English Name : *Yogurt*
Indian Name : *Dahi*

## Description

Curd or yogurt is a lactic fermentation of milk. It is esteemed for its smoothness, its pleasant and refreshing taste. It is highly versatile and health-promoting and one of the most valuable therapeutic foods.

The milk of cow is generally used in preparing yogurt in Europe and America. In India, buffalo milk is also extensively used. In Russia, the milk of sheep, goat and mare is largely used for the same purpose.

The best and purest milk should always be used for preparing the curd. Before it is curdled, the milk should be boiled for about 10 minutes and the temperature of the milk brought down to lukewarm state. Freshly cultured starter should then be added to it and mixed thoroughly with the milk. Generally one teaspoonful of starter is sufficient for every 500 ml. of milk.

The quality of curd depends to a great extent on the starter used. The better the seed the sweeter will be the aroma and firmer will be texture of the curd. In hot season the milk curdles easily. But in cold season, it is necessary to cover it with a blanket and keep it in a warm place. It generelly takes about six to eight hours for the milk to coagulate in the hot season. In cold weather it takes 12 to 16 hours for it to form a firm mass.

## Origin and History

The world yogurt is of Turkish Origin. It is believed that the first curd was made in Turkey. Legend has it that a nomad while travelling through a desert, kept some milk away in a goat-skin bag and hung it across the back of his camel. On opening the bag few hours later, he found that the liquid has been transformed into a thick tangy custard. The desert sun and the bacteria inside the bag produced the required condition for the preparation of yogurt.

Curd has played an important part in the diet of nations from time immemorial. It has been regarded as a wholesome food in India, Turkey, Egypt, Armenia, Yugoslavia, Rumania, Russia and Central Europe. In Western Europe and America also, it has become very popular during the last few decades.

**Food Value**

Curd is a very nourishing food. It is a valuable source of protein, essential vitamins and minerals. It is also a rich source of calcium and riboflavin. The proteins in curd is more readily digested than the protein in milk. It has been estimated that regular milk is only 32 per cent digested after an hour in the digestive tract, whereas 91 per cent of curd is digested within the same period of time. It is, therefore, an ideal diet for those with sensitive digestive systems, particularly young children and elderly persons.

## Curd*

| Food Value | | Minerals and Vitamins | |
|---|---|---|---|
| Moisture | 89.1% | Calcium | 149 mg |
| Protein | 3.1% | Phosphorus | 93 mg |
| Fat | 4.0% | Iron | 0.2 mg |
| Minerals | 0.8% | Vitamin A | 102 I.U. |
| Carbohydrates | 3.0% | Vitamin C | 1 mg |
| | | Small amount of Vitamin B Complex | |
| | 100% | | |

*Value per 100 gms edible portion                    **Calorific Value - 60**

## Natural Benefits and Curative Properties

Although curd has a nutritive content similar to fresh milk, it has extensive special values for therapeutic purposes. During the process of making curd, bacteria convert milk into curd and predigest milk protein. These bacteria then inhibit the growth of hostile or illness-causing bacteria inside the intestinal tract and promote beneficial bacteria needed for digestion. These friendly bacteria facilitate the absorption of minerals and aid in the synthesis of vitamins of B group. Buttermilk, which has same nutritive and curative value as curd, is prepared by churning curd and adding some water, removing the fat in the form of butter.

Curd is also considered one of the best aids to natural good looks. It supplies the nerves and the skin with healthy ingredients and counteracts the ill-effects of exposure to the scorching sun. The bacteria in curd make the skin soft and glowing. Curd mixed with orange or lemon juice is a good face cleanser. It supplies moisture to the skin and fruit juice provides the essential vitamin C. One tablespoonful of juice should be mixed in one cup of curd. This should be applied to face and neck and allowed to dry for 15 minutes. It should then be wiped of with a soft tissue and washed with water.

A mixture of oatmeal flour and yogurt has been found effective in making the skin fairer and softer. This mixture should be kept on the facial skin for 15 to 20 minutes and then washed off with warm water. For pimples, a paste of curd and Bengal gram flour or *besan* should be applied on the face and then washed off.

Curd is also considered valuable in conditioning the hair. It makes the hair soft, healthy and strong. Curd should be massaged right into the roots of the hair before being washed off. Dandruff can be removed by massaging one's hair for half an hour with curd which has been kept in the open for three days.

### Gastro-intestinal Disorders

Apart from the lactic acid organisms placed in the milk for the purpose of souring it, the acid of sour milk and its lectose content are important curative factors in a number of diseases. Curd brings relief to patients suffering from gastro-intestinal disorders such as chronic constipation and diarrhoea.

Orla Jensen of Copenhagen, author of Lactic Acid Bacteria, observes that yogurt and fermented beverages may be frequently used in case of gastric irritation where other food cannot be retained by stomach. The lactic acid, he says, is completely metabolished to carbondioxide and water is not excreted in the urine. It also does not have any effect on acid-base balance in the system. It is thus an alkaline food. Besides aiding in the digestion of food, curd decreases dryness and gas in the stomach by helping in secretion of hydrochloric acid, pepsin and renin.

The germs which give rise to infection and inflammation

such as those which cause appendicitis, diarrhoea and dysentery, cannot thrive in the presence of lactic acid found in curd and buttermilk. Beneficial results have been achieved by the use of buttermilk in the cases of colitis. Buttermilk enemas have been found beneficial in the treatment of colitis, chronic constipation, diarrhoea, dysentery, chronic appendicitis and gastric ulcer.

## Insomnia

Curd is valuable in the treatment of insomnia. The patient should take plenty of curd and massage it on the head. This will induce sleep.

## Premature Ageing

Curd has been associated with longevity. Prof. Elic Metchnikoff, a noble prize-winning Russian bacteriologist at the Pasteur Institute, believed that premature old age and decay could be prevented by taking sufficient curd in the daily diet. He made an intensive study of the problem of old age in the early 20th century. He came to the conclusion that the body is slowly being poisoned and its resistance weakened by man's normal diet and that this poisoning process could be arrested and the intestinal tract kept healthy by the constant, regular use of yogurt or some variety of acidophilus milk.

## Hepatitis and Jaundice

Excessive liberation of ammonia, which is one of the major causes of coma in hepatitis, can be prevented by liberal use of curd. The lectic acid organisms in the curd counteracts the formation of ammonia. In jaundice, curd or buttermilk sweetened with honey, makes an ideal diet.

## Burning in Rectum

Severe burning and intense itching in the rectum, after passing the stools, can be controlled and successfully treated in a couple of days by liberal use of curd and lemon juice with bland diet. Curd makes the stool acitic and alleviates the burning and itching sensations.

## Skin Disorders

The use of curd in the form of buttermilk is highly beneficial in the treatment of obstinate skin disorders such as psoriasis and eczema. The application of buttermilk compresses will also be useful in these conditions. Pads of muslin or thin cloth saturated with buttermilk may be applied to broad surface. The compresses may be worn continuously or only at night. The surface should be properly cleaned when the compress is removed. The compresses are very effective in case of skin inflammation. The intense skin irritation generally disappears quickly after the application of buttermilk compresses.

## Uses

Curd is used in numerous ways in Indian culinary art. It is eaten with both meat and vegetable curries, with rice, fruit and fish. It is eaten plain with salt and pepper, with sugar, honey, fruit, molasses and with innumerable essenses. Many dishes are cooked in curd. It is also extensively used in the form of buttermilk and *lassi*. Over 50 per cent of the total milk in the country is converted in curd.

# *Honey*

Indian Name : *Shahad*

## Description

Honey is one of nature's most splendid gifts to mankind. It possesses unique nutritional and medicinal properties. It is a viscid, saccharine substance, semi-translucent liquid of a light yellowish-brown colour. It has aromatic odour and sweet acrid taste. After some time it become opaque and crystalline. Bees alone are capable of making honey and honey comb.

The word "honey" is derived from the Arabic "han". This became 'honing' in German and 'huning' in old English. The word is used in English language as a term of endearment.

## Origin and History

In India, honey has been used for several thousand years as an ingredient for medicines. In Egypt also, it formed the basis of many medical preparations. The ancient Greeks attributed many virtues to it. Hippocrates, the father of medicine, prescribed it 2,000 years ago to his patients as a remedy for several ailments and himself also used it. He believed that honey combined with other foods was nourishing and health-giving.

Aristotle, the father of natural science, held that its use improved health and prolonged life.

It is well known that the ancient Egyptians and Greeks used honey to embalm their dead. It has a wonderful keeping quality. In a tomb of a queen of Egypt, who was buried over 3,000 years ago, was found a jar of honey which had not undergone any appreciable change in its chemical composition or in its original aroma. It has been recently found that honey retains all its qualities even after 22 years.

### Food Value

The sugars in honey are glucose, fructose and sucrose. Glucose is the simplest of the sugars. It occurs in the blood of live animals, in fruit and vegetable juices. Its restores the oxygen that is replaced by lectic and acid when fatigue sets in. Fructose, which is also known as levulose or grape sugar, crystallises more easily than. glucose and builds up tissues. Sucrose is a combination of glucose and fructose. Dextrine, which is a gummyy substance, is found in small amount in honey, but it makes honey so digestible.

Latest research indicates that the pollen in honey contains all 22 amino acids, 28 minerals, 11 enzymes. 14 fatty acids and 11 carbohydrates. Unfortunately much of these nutritive qualities are lost by heating the honey to 150⁰F for commercial use. Filtering, bottling and cooling to protects its flavour, remove the pollen grains and do not leave the honey as a pure product.

| Honey* | | | |
|---|---|---|---|
| **Food Value** | | **Minerals and Vitamins** | |
| Moisture | 20.0% | Calcium | 5 mg |
| Protein | 0.3% | Phosphorus | 16 mg |
| Minerals | 0.2% | Iron | 0.9 mg |
| Carbohydrates | 79.5% | Vitamin C | 4 mg |
| | | Small amount of | |
| | | Vitamin B Complex | |
| | 100% | | |
| *Value per 100 gms edible portion | | **Calorific Value - 319** | |

## Natural Benefits and Curative Properties

Honey is one of the finest sources of heat and energy. Energy is generated mainly by the carbohydrate foods and honey is one of the most easily digested form of carbohydrates. It enters directly into the bloodstream because of its dextrine content and this provides almost instantaneous energy. It is a boon to those with weak digestion. All organs in the body respond favourably when honey is eaten. The famous Roman physician, Galen has described honey as an all-purpose medicine for all types of diseases. It is now used as a curative and preventive for several ailments.

One spoon of fresh honey, mixed with the juice of half a lemon in a glass of lukewarm water and taken first thing in the morning, is an effective remedy for constipation and hyperacidity. Fasting on this honey-lemon juice water is highly beneficial in the treatment of obesity without loss of energy and appetite.

A mixture of honey and alcohol is believed to promote growth of hair. It is said that Japanese geisha girls, who have luxuriant hair, mix several tablespoonful of honey with alcohol, stirring them together. They massage this mixture onto the scalp, allow it to remain there for two hours and then wash or rainse with shampoo thoroughly. It is said that regular use of this honey-alcohol mixture stimulates the hair follicles to grow into luxuriant tresses.

**Heart Diseases**

Dr. Arnold Lorand, an eminent nutrition expert considers honey as the best food for the heart. He observes, "Honey is easily digested and assimilated; it is the best sweet food, as it does not cause flatulence and can prevent it to a certain extent, promoting the activity of the bowels. It can be easily added to the five meals a day I recommend in cases of arteriosclerosis and of weak hearts. As it would be unwise to leave such a hard working organ as the heart without food over the long hours of the night, I recommend heart patients to take before going to bed a glass of water with honey and lemon juice in it, and also to take it when awakening at night".[1] Honey is useful in cardiac pain and palpitation of the heart.

**Anaemia**

Honey is remarkable in building haemoglobin in the body. this is largely due to the iron, copper and manganese contained

---

1. Ibid., p. 23.

in it. It is beneficial in the treatment of anaemia as it helps maintain the right balance of haemoglobin and red blood corpuscles.

## Pulmonary Diseases

Honey is highly beneficial in the treatment of all diseases of the lungs. It is said if a jug of honey is held under the nose of an asthma patient and he inhales the air that comes into contact with the honey, he starts breathing easier and deeper. The effects last for about an hour or so. This is because honey contains a mixture of 'higher' alcohols and ethereal oil and the vapours given off by them are soothing and beneficial to the asthma patients. It usually brings relief whether the air flowing over the honey is inhaled or whether it is eaten or taken either in milk or water. Some authorities recommend one year old honey for respiratory disease.[2]

## Skin Diseases

Honey, applied externally, is considered useful in the treatment of wounds and sores. Dr. N. Zaiss, a leading Vinnese physician before the World Wars, claimed to have treated successfully thousands of cases of wounds, sores and long standing ulcers with honey. Honey, according to him soothes pain, acts as an antiseptic, hastens healing and is especially effective in curing burns and carbuncles.[3]

## Irritating Cough

The use of honey is highly beneficial in the treatment of irritating cough. As a demulcent or soothing agent, it produces a soothing effect on the inflamed mucus membrane of the upper respiratory tract and retrieves irritating cough and symptoms like difficulty in swallowing. For the same reason, it is used in the manufacture of various cough mixtures. Honey gargles are also useful in irritant cough.

## Insomnia

Honey is beneficial in the treatment of insomnia. It has hypnotic action in bringing sound sleep. It should be taken with water, before going to bed, in doses of two teaspoonfuls in a big cupful of water. Babies generally fall asleep after taking honey.

2. Ibid., p. 37.
3. Ibid., p. 35.

## Oral Diseases

Honey is valuable in keeping the mouth healthy. Applied daily over the teeth and gums, it cleans and gives sparkle to the teeth. It prevents deposit of tartar at the base of the teeth and prevents decay and early falling of the teeth. Being a mild antiseptic, it prevents the growth of harmful micro-organisms. It also keeps the gums in the healthy state, increasing their vascularity. In case of ulcers in the oral cavity, honey helps in their early healing and prevents further sepsis and pyogenic infection related bad odour and pus formation. Gargling with honey water is very useful in gingivitis due to inflammation of the gums.

## Eye Diseases

Honey is an excellent remedy for various eye ailments. Applied daily in the eyes, it improves the eye-sight. It is very useful in the treatment of itching of the eyes, trachoma, conjunctivitis and other similar diseases. Its regular internal as well as external application will prevent glaucoma in the initial stage of the disease.

Honey is valuable in the prevention of cataract formation. Two grams of onion juice and honey each, mixed together, should be kept safe in a clean bottle. It should be applied locally to the eyes with a glass rod. This is a very effective remedy for immature cataract. It resolves the already coagulated protein fibres as well as prevents further coagulation.

## Diseases of stomach

Honey is useful in maintaining the health of the stomach. It tones up the stomach, helps in proper digestion and prevents stomach diseases. It also decreases the over production of hydrochloric acid thereby preventing symptoms like nausea, vomiting and heart burn. When putrified faecal matter and undigested foods are present in the alimentary canal, honey acts as a laxative and emetic and clears the digestive canal of the waste matter.

## Old Age

Honey is specially useful in providing energy and heat to the body in old age. It dries up the phlegm and clears the system of mucus to which a person generally falls victim to in old age. One or two teaspoonful of honey in a cupful of boiling water, taken while still warm, is a refreshing and strengthening drink.

## Sexual Debility

Honey is a spermatogenic and sexual stimulant. It is regarded by many Asiatics as an aphrodisiac. They believe that it possesses a magical substance which influences the fertility of women and the virility of men. In ancient days, a simple honey potion was said to offer a feeling of rejuvenation. It was prepared by boiling three parts water to one part honey over a slow fire until two thirds remains. This honey potion is believed to promote a feeling of rejuvenation and youthful virility.[4]

# *Milk*

Indian Name : *Doodh*

## Description

Milk is one of the most common articles of food throughout the world. It occupies a unique position in the maintenance of health and healing diseases. It is considered as "Nature's most nearly perfect food."

The milk of animals has been used by mankind from time immemorial. The milk of cow, buffalow and goat is generally used. In certain places, however, milk of sheep and mare is also used. Cow's milk contains almost twice as much protein as human milk, but less sugar. Buffalow's milk contains more fat than cow's milk.

## Food Value

Milk is regarded as a complete food. It contains protein, fat, carbohydrates, all the known vitamins, various minerals and all the food ingredients considered essential for sustaining life and maintaining health. The protein of milk is of the highest biological value and it contains all the amino acids essential for body building and repair of body cells.

---

4. Carlson Wade, *Health Secrets from the Orient*, p. 208, Allied Publishers Pvt. Ltd., Bombay.

## Milk*

| Food Value | | Minerals and Vitamins | |
|---|---|---|---|
| Moisture | 87.5% | Calcium | 120 mg |
| Protein | 3.2% | Phosphorus | 90 mg |
| Fat | 4.1% | Iron | 0.2 mg |
| Minerals | 0.8% | Small amount of | |
| Carbohydrates | 4.4% | Vitamin B Complex, | |
| | | K and P | |
| | 100% | | |

*Value per 100 gms edible portion      **Calorific Value - 67**

A litre of milk provides all the calcium needed by an individual for one day, practically all the phosphorus, a liberal amount of vitamins A and C, one third or more of the protein, one eighth or more of the iron, at least one fourth of the energy, and some of vitamins B, E and D. Milk ranks high in digestibility. Its fat is 99 per cent digestible, its protein 97 per cent and its carbohydrates 98 per cent. Milk is said to require about one and a half hours for digestion. It curdles almost immediately after it reaches the stomach. The organic salts and water begin to be absorbed immediately, while the solid matters are passed on to the intestines where the fat is quickly absorbed by the lacteals.

## Natural Benefits and Curative Properties

According to Charaka, the great author of the Indian system of medicine, milk increases strength, improves memory, removes exhaustion, maintains strength and promotes long life. Experiments conducted in modern times have amply coroborated this opinion of Charaka.

Milk is the only article of diet which is well accepted as a wholesome food for persons of all ages, from infancy to old age. It is of special value in feeding infants, toddlers, growing children and expectant and nursing mothers. It is also recommended as a wholesome food for invalids.

### Under Weight

Milk diet is highly beneficial in the treatment of thinness. If one is considerably below the normal weight, the gain will be from three to five pounds a week, depending upon the quantity of milk consumed. The body gradually fills out. The eyes become clear and bright and the complexion assumes a healthy colour. The assimilative organs gain renewed energy and power and the gain in the weight is permanent.

## Poor Blood Circulation

An exclusive milk diet is very valuable for those suffering from poor blood circulation. The natural increase in circulation results from the increased amount of fluid assimilated by the stomach and intestines. Hands and feet, which are usually cold in case of poor circulation, become warm and life-like and the patient gets a feeling of well-being within a few days on the milk-diet.

## Hyperacidity

The milk diet has proved very efficacious in case of hyperacidity and other acid conditions of the stomach. It requires a large amount of acid for its digestion. As milk contains excess of alkaline forming elements, it quickly relives all acid conditions of the system.

## Insomnia

Milk is very valuable in sleeplessness. A glass of milk, sweetened with honey, should be taken every night before going to bed in this condition. It acts as a tonic and a tranquilliser. Massaging the milk over the soles of the feet has also been found effective.

## Respiratory System Disorders

Milk has proved useful in respiratory system disorders such as common cold, hoarseness laryngitis, tonsillitis, bronchitis and asthma. A glassful of pure boiled milk, mixed with a pinch of turmeric powder and few broken pepper, should be taken every night for three nights in these conditions. It will bring beneficial results.

## Skin Disorders

Cream of milk, mixed with a little vinegar and a pinch of turmeric powder, makes an effective dressing for cut wounds, other simple traumatic injuries — i.e. painful injuries and eczema. It also makes an effective poultice in ripening the blood boils and in their healing without sepsis.

## Beauty Aid

Milk is useful as a cosmetic and a beauty aids. A fresh lime should be squeezed in a glassful of boiled milk and set it for 10 minutes. It should then be applied over hands, arms, face, neck and soles in the night and allowed to dry. It should be washed with warm water in the morning. Its regular use will whiten the complexion and make the skin soft. Washing the hair with milk and egg yolk every day will promote hair growth and protect the scalp from all diseases.

# Sugarcane

Botanical Name : *Saccharum officinarum*
Indian Name : *Gannā*

## Description

Sugarcane is the most important member of the plant kingdom with a metabolism leading to the accumulation of sucrose. It is transported as glucose and fructose within the growing plant. The crop provides the cheapest of energy-giving food.

The sugarcane belongs to the grass family. It is a perennial plant which grows from 2.5 to 4.25 metres. With sufficient care, it grows upto 7.5 metres. The diametre of stems varies from 2.5 to 8 cm. It has several joints after every few centimetres.

## Origin and Distribution

The names sugar and sugarcane have been derived from the Sanskrit word, *Sharkara*. Sugercane is indigenous to India. It was cultivated here from the Vedic period and it is mentioned in some places in the ancient scriptures. Alexander the Great and his soldiers carried sugarcane from India to the west by about 325 BC. Sugarcane is now grown all over the world. India stands first in sugarcane cultivation, followed by Brazil, Cuba, China, Mexico, Pakistan, the U.S.A., South Africa and Columbia.

## Food Value

The juice is extracted from the cane by pressing it through iron rollers. It is nutritious and refreshing. It contains about 15 per cent natural sugar and is rich in organic salts and vitamins.

Originally, sugarcane was grown solely for chewing in the Pacific and South Eastern Asia, a custom which has now spread throughout most of the tropics. The juice can also be used for

## Sugarcane*

| Food Value | | Minerals and Vitamins | |
|---|---|---|---|
| Moisture | 90.2% | Calcium | 10 mg |
| Protein | - 0.1% | Phosphorus | 10 mg |
| Fat | 0.2% | Iron | 1.1 mg |
| Minerals | 0.4% | | |
| Carbohydrates | 9.1% | | |
| | 100% | | |

*Value per 100 gms edible portion          **Calorific Value - 39**

drinking or sweetening. In hot summer days, it forms a soothing drink. A little lime juice may be mixed in the juice to improve its flavour.

## Natural Benefits and Curative Properties

Sugarcane juice has many medicinal properties. It strengthens the stomach, kidneys, heart, eyes, brain and sex organs.

### Fevers

The juice is beneficial in fevers. In febrile disorders which causes fever, when there is great protein loss, liberal intake of sugarcane juice supplies the body with necessary protein and other food elements.

### Genito-urinary Disorders

Sugarcane is very useful in scanty urination. It keeps the urinary flow clear and helps the kidneys to perform their functions properly. It is also valuable in burning micturation due to high acidity, gonorrhoea, enlarged prostate, cyctitis and nepthritis. For better results, it should be mixed with lime juice, ginger juice and coconut water.

### Jaundice

Mixed with lime juice, it can hasten recovery from jaundice. It is, however, very essential that the juice, must be clean, preferably prepared at home. Resistance is low in hepatitis and any infected beverage could make matters worse.

### Weak Teeth

The juice sucked from the sugarcane can prove highly valuable in case of weak teeth due to lack of proper exercise resulting from excessive use of soft foods. It gives a form of exercise to the teeth and makes them strong. It also keeps the teeth clean and increases their life.

## Thinness

Sugarcane juice is a fattening food. It is thus an effective remedy for thinness. Rapid gain in weight can be achieved by its regular use.

## Eye Disorders

The dew which collects on the long leaves of sugarcane is useful in several eye disorders. When instilled in the eyes, it is an effective medicine in defective vision, cataract, conjunctivitis, burning of the eyes and eye-strain after excessive reading.